THE PRACTICE OF
Electrocardiography

by

Thomas M. Blake, M.D.
Professor of Medicine

University of Mississippi School of Medicine
Jackson, Mississippi

Medical Examination Publishing Co., Inc.
an Excerpta Medica company

Library of Congress Cataloging in Publication Data

Blake, Thomas Mathews, 1920-
The practice of electrocardiography.
Includes bibliographical references and index.

1. Electrocardiography.
I. Title.
RC683. 5. E5B56   616. 1'207547   80-13084
ISBN 0-87488-903-0 hard cover
ISBN 0-87488-997-9 paperback

SIMULTANEOUSLY PUBLISHED IN:

Europe : HANS HUBER PUBLISHERS
              Bern, Switzerland

Japan   : IGAKU-SHOIN Ltd.
              Tokyo, Japan

Contents

PREFACE

BASIC CONSIDERATIONS

    I   Introduction 1
   II   Electrocardiography in Perspective 5
  III   Anatomic and Physiologic Basis of the
         Electrocardiogram 12
   IV   Reference Frames 22
    V   The Normal Electrocardiogram 44

MECHANISM

   VI   Impulse Formation and Conduction 49
  VII   Disorders of Impulse Formation 56
 VIII   Abnormalities of AV Conduction 76
   IX   Disorders of Intraventricular Conduction 85

STRUCTURE AND FUNCTION

    X   Structure and Function 98
   XI   Abnormalities of Repolarization 103
  XII   Myocardial Infarction 113
 XIII   Chamber Imbalance 123

MISCELLANY

  XIV   Methods 135
  XV   Miscellany 149
 XVI   Description and Interpretation of the Tracing 168
        References 186
        Index 229

Preface

Learning, if it is to lead to understanding, must proceed from a base of information shared by student and instructor; otherwise there is a risk that the student will end up knowing words and "facts" but understanding little. The text that follows is designed for readers whose information base includes an elementary knowledge of anatomy, physiology, and electricity, a group that includes doctors, medical and nursing students, and many technicians. Those whose knowledge is more than elementary need spend very little time on the first few chapters, while those who have had little instruction in these subjects will find there much of what they need to know. The information in later chapters is related directly to electrocardiography and should be enough to enable the student to describe a tracing and reach a reasonable interpretation in most cases; references to the literature are provided for those who want to go into the subject more deeply. Doctors whose EKG experience is based on pattern recognition and who are accustomed to accepting generalizations and disclaimers in their interpretation may be surprised by the order of the approach offered here, and also may enjoy it. Medical students, for whom the book is intended primarily, and nursing students can expect to build a firm foundation in a subject they will use the rest of their lives, and technicians can learn to describe a tracing, extract a diagnosis from it in many instances, and, especially, to understand better the importance of the work they are doing. All three of these groups should find something to help in their work with electrocardiograms—and that is the object of the book.

Logical organization of the subject matter is easy in principle but impossible in detail; the wish to present information in an orderly fashion, beginning with anatomy and physiology and proceeding to application, is often in conflict with the need to make it useful and available, to apply something that logically might not have been discussed yet. Resolution of this conflict is sometimes arbitrary. The presentation begins with Galvani and his recognition of bioelectricity and ends with an EKG interpretation ready for translation to orders on the patient's chart. It is not expected, however, that many readers will begin with page one and go straight through to the end of the book, and organization has been modified with the intent of making each segment useful as a unit with connections to other sections provided by cross references. Many, perhaps most, readers will work with the last chapter first and it is hoped that references there to earlier chapters will lead them through the whole book sooner or later and that they will follow the directions to the literature that are offered. Most of the references have been chosen because of their readily availability, current status, and/or because of their bibliographies; only a few are classics and there has been no attempt at comprehensiveness.

The writing is intended to express ideas as precisely as possible in appropriately basic language, emphasizing at every opportunity the importance of distinguishing between what one knows and how he knows it, what he thinks and why he thinks it, between reporting and interpretation (571). As many components as possible are identified in the analysis of each problem even though they may be discarded later during the synthetic process when a diagnosis is being prepared. Jargon is kept to a minimum and new terms are defined as they are introduced. Redundancy is avoided, but repetition for effect or convenience is utilized; sometimes the same thought is expressed in different words in different portions of the book.

Policies governing the presentation of information and the processing of a tracing can be summarized by the following guidelines. These describe an order of thinking that the reader knows already, but experience teaches that they are often disregarded.

Analysis

(1) Identify as many components of each problem, each tracing, as possible.

(2) Describe each component in appropriate detail, distinguishing clearly between description and interpretation; i.e., between what one sees and what he thinks it means.

Synthesis

(3) Re-assemble all the data into a diagnosis; i.e., a statement of

what can be said with confidence about mechanism, structure, and function.

(4) Speculate beyond the factual to the degree appropriate in the circumstances. That a component of a tracing cannot be digitized does not diminish its reality or its importance but requires that the interpreter realize that its evaluation depends on judgment, the art of medicine; it is important to localize the interface between what is known and what is speculative.

(5) Present the diagnosis in terms that will be understood by the doctor to whom it is directed. The product of an EKG interpretation is an expression of professional opinion that will be incorporated into plans for the care of a patient. It must be as precise and unambiguous as possible and its composition requires the responsible use of language.

(6) Explanatory comment, discussion, or consultative opinion may be added as needed, but this must be kept separate from the diagnosis which tells what information is to be had from the tracing itself. In each of these steps decisions must be made, decisions that have the potential for influencing the well-being of the patient, and the basis for each of them, the alternatives among which one chooses, must be identified and evaluated.

A consequence of experience in describing and interpreting electrocardiograms is that one develops both speed and confidence, but speed without accuracy and without understanding of what one is doing is of no value to anyone and is certainly not a measure of professional attainment. The aim is understanding and clinical usefulness, not speed.

This book, although substantially new, is a logical derivative of its author's *Introduction to Electrocardiography,* the last edition of which was published by Appleton-Century-Crofts in 1972. The title has been changed not only to indicate the extent of the present work's originality, but also to emphasize one of its principal reasons for being: the forceful expression of the position that to interpret an electrocardiogram is to practice medicine. The views expressed have been developed with the help of many, many medical students, house officers, practicing doctors, and technicians and would not ever have been set down in writing without the stimulus provided by daily sessions with them. Portions of the manuscript for this version have been read by Drs. George Burch, James R. Galyean, Harper K. Hellems, Edgar Hull, Thomas N. James, Patrick H. Lehan, Angel K.

Markov, Gaston Rodriquez, Isadore Rosenfeld, and M.P. Smith, Jr. None of these agreed with everything he read and none is responsible for what has finally appeared in print, but all helped and I am grateful to them. Special appreciation must be expressed to Mrs. Jocelyn B. Milton for her typing and forbearance and to all of the other typists in the Heart Station.

Thomas M. Blake, M.D.
Professor of Medicine
University of Mississippi School of Medicine
Jackson, Mississippi

notice

The editor(s) and/or author(s) and the publisher of this book have made every effort to ensure that all therapeutic modalities that are recommended are in accordance with accepted standards at the time of publication.

The drugs specified within this book may not have specific approval by the Food and Drug Administration in regard to the indications and dosages that are recommended by the editor(s) and/or author(s). The manufacturer's package insert is the best source of current prescribing information.

CHAPTER I

Introduction

Students beginning their clinical work seem to see electrocardiograms as something new and different; they know the language of the method but have difficulty relating tracings to the fundamentals of structure and function they have spent so much time learning. Real study of electrocardiography is deferred in most cases until relatively late in residency training by which time the young doctor, having used EKG reports empirically for so long, may not be motivated to review the basic sciences or to question tradition. A major intent of this book is to encourage the student to begin early in his clinical experience to deal with the electrocardiogram as an understandable application of what he knows about cardiac structure and function and to help him utilize it as effectively as possible in the care of patients. Most readers will not become electrocardiographers, but all will deal with EKGs one way or another and must know when and why they can be expected to be useful and to recognize the possibility that misinterpretation may harm the patient.

A surgeon faced with a difficult operation must know a great deal about anatomy, physiology, biochemistry, physics, pharmacology, and other fundamentals in order to be able to perform that procedure, say a cholecystectomy, satisfactorily. To the uninformed observer it may seem that technique, the manual dexterity that comes with experience, is all that counts. Such an observer might conclude that to learn to do cholecystectomies all one would have to do would be to watch a few, help in a few, and then do them himself; and it is possible that such an approach might work some of the time, perhaps even often, but no one in his right mind would actually attempt such a thing, much less submit to it in the role of patient. Something might go wrong, and the purely technically trained

1

surgeon would be at a loss as to what to do. The resulting catastrophe would be obvious to all very quickly, and the surgeon would not have many more patients.

The interpretation of electrocardiograms calls for similar preparation and understanding, but many doctors who have had good instruction in basic sciences and considerable success in clinical experience still treat an electrocardiogram as just so many lines on a piece of graph paper to be "read" by memorizing a few patterns and fitting the complexes at hand into one of them in a manner that is sometimes procrustean. If a mistake is made it does not produce pain, bleeding, or sudden death, and neither doctor nor patient may even be aware of the error. The patient's life, though, may be modified so as to lessen at least his happiness, and often his productivity, if not his longevity. Some may depend upon consultants for interpretation of tracings, and this can be a satisfactory arrangement if they know what sort of information to expect from the study and provide the interpreter with pertinent clinical data. If the interpreter hides behind disclaimers such as "compatible with" and "not inconsistent with the possibility of," however, and the doctor, failing to recognize the uncertainty implicit in these expressions, thinks a diagnosis has been made, the patient may suffer. To accept a computer readout as the answer without exercising professional judgment shows lack of understanding of what the computer is supposed to do and puts the patient at unnecessary risk.

All this is meant to say that if one is to use electrocardiography he must know something about it, whether he interprets his own tracings or not. It is to this end that the subject will be dealt with here. It will be presented briefly enough so that the student will be able to get the big picture without becoming lost in detail, but enough factual information will be included to permit useful interpretation of most tracings, and the serious student will be guided to the literature.

The following is from a summary of an article by Dr. Frank Wilson[1] entitled "Interpretation of the Ventricular Complex of the Electrocardiogram." It was published in 1947 and is just as pertinent today as it was then.

We shall not attempt a long discussion of the present wretched state of electrocardiographic diagnosis or the misery attributable to it. The errors made in this field are due in large measure to the same human frailties that are responsible for errors in others, medical and non-medical. We wish, however, to make a few comments which appear to us worthwhile. In our opinion, no physician should refer a patient to another for an electrocardiographic examination and report without giving the referee a resume of the data which he has collected (if he has any) nor without letting him know exactly what information the electrocardiographic examination is expected to yield.

We think also that there are altogether too many physicians who want to, and try to, read electrocardiograms, but are unwilling to go back to the fundamental principles upon which the interpretation of the electrocardiograms must be based. In our opinion, it is impossible to use diagnostic criteria intelligently unless they are fundamentally sound and the foundations on which they rest are clearly understood by the user. . . .

Electrocardiography is one of the most exact of diagnostic methods. Its potential value is great, but it is not being used to the best advantage. Electrocardiographic abnormalities are not diseases. They have no important bearing upon life expectancy of the patient, or the extent to which his mode of life should be altered when there is reasonable doubt as to the nature of the factor or factors responsible for them in that particular case.

Dr. Tinsley Harrison[2] said of this advice:

If electrocardiography were practiced according to the philosophy expounded above, and if the medical profession were aware of the limitations as well as the value of electrocardiography, there would be fewer patients leading miserable and unnecessarily restricted lives as the result of harmful and unwarranted interpretations of electro-cardiographic records.

Another pertinent observation is that of Dr. William Bennett Bean:[3]

The less experience one has with a laboratory procedure the more confidence he has in its precision.

Electrocardiography is in many respects an isolated technique whose disciplines are of little interest to workers in other fields.[4] Its basis in anatomy, physiology, physics, and other relatively objective sciences is well-founded, but in application it remains almost completely clinical; usefulness to the patient is the only measure of its accuracy and value — and this is determined to a large extent by the doctor. Disorders of mechanism can almost always be described in more than one way, for instance, and there is no way to prove, at autopsy or otherwise, exactly which one is correct. Evaluation of even anatomic change in the ventricular myocardium is extremely limited by the need for complex techniques of study that are not applied very often,[5-7] and quantitative definitions of hypertrophy, dilatation, and even infarction are subject to wide variation. Proof of functional changes such as strain, metabolic imbalance, and drug toxicity is based entirely on clinical evidence. Normal is difficult to define closely,[8-10] and the limitations of the method include wide intra-observer and inter-observer variations.[11,12] The importance of the words chosen to express the findings in a tracing cannot be over-emphasized.[13] The principal justification for making most routine tracings is their potential value as controls, and even this benefit is so tenuous that its cost may be hard to justify. The electrocardiogram by itself is rarely definitive in the decision-making process.

Sir William Osler said that to see patients without books is to sail an uncharted sea and that to see books without patients is never to have gone to sea at all; electrocardiograms could be substituted for patients in this statement. A few exemplary tracings are included in this edition, but the book is intended for use by students working with real, fresh, uninterpreted tracings, i.e., patients, preferably under the supervision of an experienced electrocardiographer. It is a lab manual, not an atlas. Collateral reading in other texts, not necessarily new, will be helpful; all have something to offer, and sometimes students learn better from one approach than another.

CHAPTER II

Electrocardiography in Perspective

It is appropriate at the beginning of a study that the subject be defined clearly and its position and relative importance in the scheme of things indentified. This chapter is designed to do this for electrocardiography by introducing some of its basic terminology and concepts and by reviewing its development in the changing reference frame of clinical medicine.

An electrocardiogram is a record of the electrical activity of the heart, a graph of voltage against time. The instrument that makes the record is called an electrocardiograph, EKG machine, or cart, and the record itself a tracing, ECG, or EKG.* The nomenclature and appearance of EKGs are so well known that we sometimes forget that tracings are at best only representations of electrical events, symbols, and it may take conscious effort to realize that a symbol is not the thing symbolized.[571]

As a clinical discipline electrocardiography is closely comparable to pathology and radiology; the practitioner in each case is a consultant the product of whose efforts is a message to another doctor. But there are differences. When a pathologist looks at a tissue section through a microscope, he examines the real thing itself, tissue, a piece of the patient, and a radiologist studying a chest film looks at a picture of a real thing. Electrical forces generated in the heart are real, too, of course, but more abstract than tissue and pictures, and the electrocardiographer deals with only a diagram of their mean values for each instant in time. Nonetheless, electro-

---

*ECG is logical as an abbreviation of the English word as well as of its three Latin components, but the word itself began in German (Elektrokardiogramm) and EKG is the traditional abbreviation that will be used in this book.

cardiography ranks with history, physical examination, and x-ray as a fundamental method of examination of the heart and is applicable at some time or other to nearly everybody. Its immediate value is very small in most cases but very great in some.

Bioelectricity has been known at least since Galvani observed the effects of electrical current on frogs' legs nearly two hundred years ago, and electrical activity has been noted in association with the heartbeat since 1856, but electrocardiography is usually dated from 1887 and the work of Augustus D. Waller. Dr. Waller, son of the English physiologist who described degeneration of nerve, was born in Paris, educated in Scotland, and worked in England. He had a long and illustrious career but is remembered best for demonstrating that the electrical activity associated with the heartbeat can be recorded without opening the thorax and that it precedes mechanical activity. He used a capillary electrometer in his experiments, a glass tube containing sulfuric acid and dipping into a reservoir of mercury. The two components of this system were connected to the body and, when the electrical field between them changed, their interface fluctuated; a light source caused the mercury column to cast a shadow on a moving photographic plate — and the first human electrocardiogram was recorded.[24]

At the same time that Waller was working in London, another young man, a 27-year-old physiologist named Willem Einthoven, had begun his investigations of the same subject across the North Sea at the University of Leyden in Holland. He was dissatisfied with the response characteristics of the capillary electrometer, and in 1903 published a description[25] of a much more sensitive instrument capable of recording clearly and accurately from the surface of the body the changes in electrical potential associated with the heartbeat. Einthoven's "string" galvanometer* was a radical improvement over earlier instruments. Its principle was simple: a movable indicator suspended in the constant electrical field between the poles of a magnet will change its position when a difference in potential between its two ends causes current to flow through it and the magnetic field around it to fluctuate proportionately. Dr. Einthoven used a "string" of quartz plated with gold or platinum as an indicator, or meter. The ends were attached to the body and fluctuation in

---

*A galvanometer is a device for measuring electricity.

electrical potential within the heart produced tiny deflections of the string that were recorded on moving photographic film as a shadow in a beam of light. Electronic amplification and more effective recording systems have evolved, but the basic concept introduced by Einthoven is still the heart of all EKG machines.

Professor Einthoven also identified the anatomic and physiologic characteristics of the body that govern the distribution of electrical signals at its surface, are approximately constant, and can be assumed to be true in humans generally, Einthoven's premises. These are the rules by which tracings are interpreted and which are summarized as "Einthoven's triangle" (see page 26). He named the deflections, too. In publications of early tracings made with capillary electrometers, the deflections were designated A, B, C, and D, but the labels P, Q, R, S, T, and U[26,570] were favored by Einthoven and, except for an early period of controversy, have been used ever since.

By 1910 or thereabouts, both the instrument for making tracings and the rules for interpreting them were available. The method was thought of at first as a laboratory gadget for use by physiologists, but it was not long before its potential for the diagnosis of disease was recognized, and the first man associated prominently with its clinical application was Sir Thomas Lewis. Dr. Lewis, who corresponded with Einthoven and cooperated with the Cambridge Instrument Company in the development of methods and their application, was interested chiefly in disorders of impulse formation and conduction. He indentified many principles that are the basis for modern practice, contrived much of the terminology, and is known best by today's medical students because of his concept of "circus conduction" as an explanation for what we know as atrial fibrillation and what before than had been called rebellious palpitations, chaos cordis, or delirium cordis.

Electrocardiographers continued for a long time to be concerned almost entirely with the formation and conduction of impulses, and one reason for this was that so little was known of diseases affecting the structure and function of the heart. That there might be such a clinical entity as myocardial infarction had been considered in the late 19th century, but its recognition as an event that one could survive dates from 1912 and the classic paper of Dr. James B. Herrick of Chicago. When the observations recorded in this paper were presented to the Association of American Physicians, they aroused almost no interest at all and went over "like a dud."[561] Dr. Herrick's interest continued, though, and in 1917 he saw a 37-year-old doctor with chest pain, made an electrocardiogram that showed ST-T characteristics similar to those that had been demonstrated recently in dogs following ligation of a coronary artery;[562] thus began the use of the electrocardiogram for the diagnosis of myocardial infarction.

The ability of quinine to restore sinus mechanism in patients with atrial fibrillation had been noted by Wenckebach,[576] and in 1918, Frey introduced quinidine, an optical isomer of quinine and still the prototype of antiarrhythmic agents, as more effective for this purpose.

By 1920, then, myocardial infarction could be diagnosed, it was possible to identify the disorders of impulse formation and conduction that may be associated with it, and potent antiarrhythmic therapy was available, but electrocardiographs were not widely available, only leads 1, 2, and 3 were in use, and prominent cardiologists could present logical reasons to question the usefulness of the EKG in its diagnosis.[575] Texts published as late as the 1930s said almost nothing about myocardial infarction, and it was not until the early forties that its diagnosis became widespread.

Einthoven's original three leads (page 26) were useful for study of forces in the frontal plane only, and in 1932 Wolferth and Wood[28] suggested the use of a posteroanterior lead, lead IV, made by placing the left arm electrode on the back and the one from the right arm over the precordium and turning the selector switch to lead I. This made a tracing very similar to modern mid-precordial leads but with the polarity reversed. A modification, lead IVF, utilized the left arm electrode at the apex and the right arm electrode on the left leg to produce a curve with the polarity used now, but its accuracy and reproducibility were limited by the problem of defining the location of the apex. In the same year, Dr. Frank N. Wilson and his group[29] published their first description of a central terminal of zero potential, the basis for the V leads and three dimensional electrocardiography, and the next few years saw a rapidly changing series of theories and lead systems. In 1938, the American Heart Association and the Cardiac Society of Great Britian and Ireland[30] did much to bring order to the field by agreeing on six positions for the chest electrode (C) defined in terms of easily identifiable landmarks of the bony thorax and eliminating the need for locating the apex (see page 27). The same group agreed that the polarity of leads developed after the original three should be standardized with the "exploring" electrode positive. The position of the positive electrode determines the name of the lead, and a positive deflection means that the process of depolarization is approaching that electrode. IVF was replaced by leading from the several precordial positions to the right arm (CR), the left arm (CL), the left leg (CF), or Wilson's central terminal (V) (see page 27). There were differences of opinion as to the relative merits of these systems but by the mid-1940s V leads were standard. Goldberger's "augmented" V leads followed very shortly (see page 30), and the lead system, in a state of flux for fifteen years, became stable and has not changed since.

Limitation of the usefulness of a mean value plotted against time, a scalar presentation, was recognized early by theorists working with electrocardiography, and in 1920 Mann projected the information from two leads on a plane in a single figure that he called a monocardiogram.[55,573] With development of the cathode ray oscilloscope in the 1920s,[574] it became possible to write this figure directly on the screen, a vectorcardiogram (VCG)*, but hopes that substantial information not available in the scalar tracing could be had from the vectorcardiogram proved to be unfounded; both versions, scalar and vector, contain the same information. The value of vectorcardiography has been largely as a means of permitting better understanding of the interrelations of the 12 views, or leads, of the more convenient scalar tracing. A factor in the relatively small application it has in clinical medicine is that no reference frame for it has been accepted as standard. An equilateral tetrahedron would be a logical extension of Einthoven's triangle, but Einthoven's premises are not applicable in the posteroanterior dimension. The Frank system of leads[477] is used probably more than any other, but it has many modifications. There is no truly orthogonal system for electrocardiography, either scalar or vector, but leads 1 and aVF (X and Y) are mutually perpendicular and define a frontal plane and, for practical purposes and within the clinical limits of the method, V_1 serves effectively as a PA, or Z, lead.

The extreme sensitivity of the early string galvanometer that

---

*A scalar value has only magnitude and can be represented completely by a point on a line; a vector value, both direction and magnitude and is represented by a line.

made it capable of recording tracings in the first place also made it a very difficult instrument to handle. Amplifiers and better recorders were produced during the twenties and thirties, but these machines, too, were delicate, complicated, and expensive, and the processing of exposed film was necessary before the tracing could be seen. In the 1940s stable and dependable direct-writing systems were introduced for the first time and, though there was some resistance to them on theoretically valid grounds, they soon replaced photographic methods. The most effective of these, a heated stylus writing on a knife-edge over which heat-sensitive paper is drawn tightly, is still widely used (see page 142).

The technical capacity for making electrocardiograms at a distance had been present from the beginning, Einthoven himself having recorded tracings from patients in a hospital a mile from his laboratory, but there had been little need for it. In the 1950s when means for the electrical control of cardiac activity, pacing and defibrillation, became available, tele-electrocardiography became useful, a profusion of monitoring devices appeared promptly, and the coronary care unit came into being.

By 1950, good electrocardiograms were available to any doctor and any patient anywhere at low cost but methods for extraction and interpretation of the information they contained had not kept pace with technologic advance. At about this time Dr. Robert P. Grant, a major figure in modern electrocardiography, put some of the most basic concepts of analysis into terms that could be understood by ordinary doctors, emphasizing the importance of the spatial interrelationship of the components of the tracing by a process that he called "vector analysis." Up to that time, tracings had been "read" on the basis of memorized numbers and patterns with little order, logic, or reasoning. Dr. Grant's text changed this and is necessary reading for any serious student of the subject.[14]

While all these advances in understanding and instrumentation were being introduced, interpretation of tracings by methods that had been used since the beginning of the century continued. Qualified doctors were few, and the "reading" of EKGs was a small component of their work; detailed analysis of the curves, necessary for secure interpretation, was simply too time-consuming to be practical. With the advent of the digital computer in the 1960s this conflict between what should be done and what could be done began to be resolved. Machines can be classified as "prosthetic," those that do only what man can do but do it faster or better, and "autonomous," those that can do things that man cannot do under any circumstances as, for instance, a clock.[572] A digital computer is a prosthetic machine, in this sense, and anolog data such as those in scalar electrocardiograms are ideally suited for digitization and manipulation by it, i.e., the computer, a machine, can be made to do the time-consuming, tedious "scut work" while man's brain is used for thinking, for making decisions. Introduction of the digital computer into the practice of electrocardiography was a tremendous advance and still has not seen its most effective application (see page 157).

What of the future? Analysis of names that have been applied to records of the electrical activity of the heart can be used as a basis for prediction. Einthoven called the graph he produced an elektrokardiogramm, EKG, failing to take into account that it would not be the only form in which this information might be presented. The E of EKG has been subdivided; to differentiate between a vectorcardiogram and an electrocardiogram is not etymologically appropriate — they are at different levels of abstraction; logically, distinction would be between a vectorcardiogram (VCG) and a scalarcardiogram (SCG). Both are electrocardiograms and both expressions of a series of mean values, inscriptions made by a device that indicates only a single *point* at a time and differing only in the graphic presentation of that point. Even when the data from planes perpendicular to each other are correlated and a three-dimensional loop is constructed, the information still shows only the net result of all the forces at work at any given instant. It is like describing a tug-of-war in terms of only the flag in the center without showing the opposing forces.

At least in theory, the future must hold a holocardiogram. Holography,[486] an important new method of presenting information, combines laser and photographic methods to produce three-dimensional images that can be viewed from any angle much as a sculpture. To produce a holo-electrocardiogram would require a technique for adapting the electrical energy available at the surface of the body for reproduction by holographic methods. This has not been done yet, but it is tempting to predict the result: the holographic representation of the process of depolarization as it traverses the ventricular myocardium from endocardium to epicardium would be a sort of three-dimensional figure that could show, literally, electrical holes in the heart.

CHAPTER III

Anatomic and Physiologic Basis of the Electrocardiogram

By the time medical students have advanced to clinical work and are ready to use information taken from electrocardiograms in the care of patients, they will have forgotten some of the anatomy and physiology needed for extracting and evaluating that information. A brief review of these subjects is presented here.

Anatomy

The *sinus node,* a structure defined only vaguely in the morphologic sense, is an aggregation of specialized tissue in the right atrial wall near the superior vena cava[536] (Figure 3-1). Under the control of humoral and neural influences, it originates electrical impulses more or less regularly at rates between about 30 or 40 and over 200 a minute. There are at least three specialized internodal pathways by way of which these impulses may be conducted preferentially through the atria (the tracts of Bachman, Thorel, and Wenckebach), and interatrial pathways have been described, too, but all these are ill-defined.[33-36,462] For most useful purposes, depolarization may be considered to proceed centrifugally from the sinus node at a rate of about 1,000 mm per second,[40] arriving ultimately at the atrioventricular (AV) node, the only electrical pathway into the ventricles in the normal heart.

Until surprisingly recently the *AV node* was more of a concept than an anatomic reality for most doctors; few medical students having finished a course in anatomy could say that they had seen one. It was so real from an electrophysiologic point of view, though, and

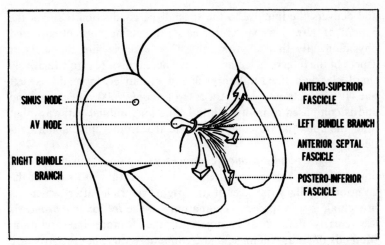

Figure 3-1. Schematic representation of intracardiac conduction. The signal may be considered as spreading over the atria from the sinus node in a manner similar to radiation of ripples from a stone dropped in a pond. It enters the ventricles through the AV junctional area, traverses the bundle of His, is distributed to the subendocardial aspect of the ventricular myocardium through its subdivisions, and spreads outward through the walls in a radial fashion. The right bundle branch is a relatively uncomplicated structure without major subdivisions; the left is much more complex, branching diffusely.

with the advent of intracardiac surgery it assumed such increased practical significance, that it became the subject of much study. Its anatomy and blood supply have been described in detail and its electrophysiologic characteristics have been explored extensively.[36-38,40] It has been described as pale in color, ovoid, about 5 mm long, and located subendocardially in the base of the interatrial septum near the coronary sinus. There may or may not exist another collection of tissue with inherent automaticity just proximal to it, the *coronary sinus node.*

In the proximal portion of the AV node the impulse is slowed to a rate as low as 20 mm per second. Within the node itself there may be more than one longitudinal pathway through which electrical wavefronts may progress at different rates under different circumstances, but in normals the tissue functions as a single electrical channel[33,412] and delivers the impulse to the specialized conduction tissue of the *bundle of His*. This structure, easier to define conceptually and physiologically than anatomically,[412,507] extends into the superior aspect of the interventricular septum where it divides into a relatively small, clearly defined right branch and a relatively large, diffuse left one. It conducts impulses at a rate of about 1,000 mm per second and is composed of multiple interlacing longitudinal pathways that offer the potential for complicated electrocardiographic abnormalities.

The *right bundle branch* continues as a thin, undivided strand down the right side of the interventricular septum to its end at the anterior papillary muscle of the right ventricle after which its branching is widespread. The anatomy of the *left bundle branch* is less clearly defined and subject to much more interpretation. Methods of study, findings, and terminology vary, but the structure seems to have more of the characteristics of a frayed cable than the right bundle branch, which is like a single strand or wire. Early in its course, in the subendocardial aspect of the left side of the interventricular septum just beneath the aortic valve, it divides into more or less well-defined groups, or fascicles, of fibers the description and classification of which are controversial, there being some question as to whether the subdivisions (posteroinferior, anterosuperior, and central or septal) are functionally distinct. Most attention has been devoted to the anterosuperior distribution (see page 89).

The first part of the ventricular myocardium to be depolarized is the left side of the interventricular septum, the impulse reaching its upper third via the anterior division of the left bundle branch and the middle and lower thirds via the posterior division.[43] The impulse is delivered to the right side of the septum at the same time as the left, but the component of the septum derived embryologically from the left ventricle is so much greater than that related to the right that the result is as if a single force had originated on the left and moved anteriorly and to the right. The rate of propagation of depolarization in this specialized conduction tissue is so great that the impulse is delivered effectively simultaneously to the subendocardium of both ventricles. From here it proceeds outward at rates as great as 4,000 mm per second via the *Purkinje network* with which the subdivisions of the His bundle merge and which communicates in some manner with the ventricular myocardium.[41] Within the myocardium the conduction velocity is slower, on the order of 400 mm per second. The net, or mean, value of this complex process is directed first toward the apex, then to the left, posteriorly, and downward, and, finally, upward toward the base of the heart, dorsad, and a bit to the right.[44]

Repolarization must follow before the cycle can be repeated. Repolarization of the atria is not detectable in the normal electrocardiogram, but ventricular repolarization is responsible for a major part of the information contained in the tracing.

Electrophysiology

It is a characteristic of living muscle to be polarized; that is, its cells may be thought of as surrounded by a membrane and covered with positively charged ions on the outside, each in equilibrium with a negatively charged one on the inside. In this resting state, the cell is in electrical balance, and no difference of potential can be recognized by a galvanometer, both of whose electrodes are outside it. When a stimulus results in permeability of the membrane so that ions can cross it, depolarization occurs. In normal muscle, restoration of the polarized state, repolarization, follows, and so on. It is the process of depolarization that provides the electrical stimulus for mechanical contraction and is responsible for the P wave and QRS of the electrocardiogram; the ST-T complex and the U wave are written during repolarization.

A few diagrams can help (Figure 3-2). Let us picture a strip of cardiac muscle in a volume conductor filled with physiologic saline. (A volume conductor is one in which electrical impulses are conducted in all directions instead of along a single course as in a linear conductor such as a wire.) The muscle is polarized, its outer surface covered with positive ions, and is observed from a truly unipolar electrode attached to the positive pole of a galvanometer whose negative pole is at infinity. In the *resting* or *polarized* state, no difference of potential is apparent, and the galvanometer indicates nothing. If the membrane is rendered permeable to electrical charges at the end of the strip farthest from the electrode, polarity cannot be maintained, and a wave of *depolarization*, a *boundary of potential difference*, progresses rapidly away from this point with its leading edge polarized, positive, and its trailing edge depolarized, negative. As this boundary approaches the exploring electrode, the galvanometer registers increasing positivity, an upstroke.

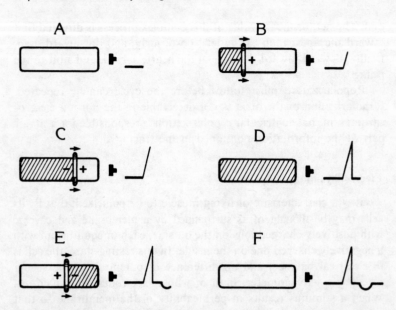

Figure 3-2. Depolarization and repolarization of a hypothetical muscle strip. In A the resting strip in a volume conductor is observed from the positive pole of a unipolar lead indicated by the electrode at the right. The tissue is polarized (positive on the outside and negative on the inside), but the membrane is intact, the outside electrode "sees" no difference in potential in the system, and the galvanometer records no deflection. When depolarization begins at the left of the strip, B, an unstable condition exists with part of the tissue polarized and part of it not. A boundary of potential difference describes the interface between the two sections, and this moves rapidly to the right, C. This process is recorded as a deflection of the stylus; the instrument is wired so that the deflection is positive when the electrode faces the positive side of the boundary. D shows depolarization completed; there is no difference of potential in the system, and the trace has returned to the baseline. In E the relatively slow process of repolarization has begun at the point that was depolarized first, and, with the electrode facing the negative side of the developing difference in potential, a downstroke is written. In F the cycle has been completed, and the trace is back to the baseline. In the ideal strip the areas under the curves are equal and of opposite sign.

When the whole muscle strip has been depolarized, no potential difference exists in the system and the pointer returns to the mid-position or baseline. Soon the process of repolarization begins — in the hypothetical circumstances described here it will be at the same point at which depolarization had begun, though in the heart, the process is much more complex.[45] The boundary of potential difference resulting from the relatively slow process of repolarization is the reverse of that which characterized depolarization; its negative side faces the electrode, and a negative deflection is recorded. The total energy generated during repolarization equals that expended during depolarization, so the areas subtended by the two curves are equal but their signs are opposite. In the hypothetical muscle strip under these ideal conditions the T wave is negative when the QRS is positive, but in the normal electrocardiogram this is not the case.

Depolarization may be compared to discharge of a condenser, an abrupt, passive process representing release of potential built up during repolarization. This relatively massive event is not easily influenced by small biochemical or other physiologic changes and some major modification, almost always structural, is required to alter it. Repolarization, on the other hand, is an active process, a build-up comparable to the charging of a condenser. It involves small potentials acting over a longer period in different areas of the myocardium at the same time and may be changed easily by almost any influence — temperature, pressure, biochemical and enzymatic processes, and other variables.

When susceptibility to repolarization is influenced by something other than the normal refractory period, changes in pressure for instance, the process is modified. If we postulate a gradient from the left of the strip to the right (Figure 3-3), it may be seen that even though the refractory period will be complete at the left end first, repolarization will be retarded here by the greater pressure and must begin somewhere else, at the end nearer the electrode in this instance. Such a course of events will result in a T wave (repolarization) of the same sign as the QRS (depolarization) because the electrode faces the positive side of the boundary of potential difference during repolarization as well as during depolarization. The diagram shows nice, smooth curves, and the gradient indicated is a simple, uncomplicated one, but in the myocardium of the beating heart there are multiple gradients from endocardium to epicardium, gradients of

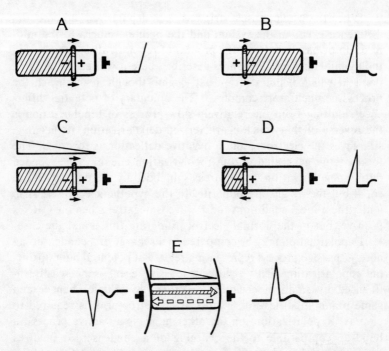

Figure 3-3. Effect of transmyocardial gradient. In A depolarization of a muscle strip proceeds toward the positive electrode writing an upstroke. In B depolarization has been completed, and repolarization is occurring; having begun at the point that was depolarized first, it proceeds in the same direction as depolarization, but now the electrode faces the negative side of the boundary of potential difference, and a negative deflection appears. A functional gradient between the ends of the strip, due to differences in pressure of other features, as indicated in C, has no detectable effect on depolarization but modifies repolarization, D, reversing its direction in this example, so that it causes a positive deflection to be written. Conditions in the ventricular wall are similar to those in the muscle strip in D. The curve on the left, E, represents the view from the inner aspect of the free wall of the left ventricle (closely comparable to clinical aVR); that on the right shows the same events seen from the opposite side (V₆).

oxygen, lactic acid, temperature, and pressure, for instance; the course of repolarization is influenced by all of them, and the result is very similar to that indicated here.

Imagine that the muscle strip represents a segment of the free wall of the left ventricle as proposed in the figure. Depolarization is from endocardium to epicardium (solid arrow) and repolarization in the opposite direction (dotted arrow). This is probably a fairly good representation of the type of thing that actually takes place. Repolarization begins during ventricular systole while there is an endocardial-epicardial pressure gradient that influences coronary blood flow, and transient differentials in the concentration of metabolites and oxygen must exist between one part of the myocardium and another.[405] Add the fact that this is taking place in three-dimensional space, and remember that information in any lead represents the net result of all this projected as a single point on that lead, and it is not difficult to understand that the curve written during ventricular repolarization, the T wave, in the normal electrocardiogram is at least different from that in the hypothetical muscle strip. In the normal human electrocardiogram, T is of the same sign as QRS in most views (leads), which is to say that the forces generated during repolarization are oriented in very nearly the same direction as those of depolarization, a finding nearly the opposite of that in the hypothetical muscle strip. Their areas, though, are not exactly equal. They can be measured and expressed in millivolt-seconds, and the relation between them can be indicated by a vector on the triaxial reference system (page 27). This relationship between the two processes is called the *ventricular gradient,* an indication of the degree of departure from ideal. Rarely measured and used as such in day-to-day interpretation of electrocardiograms, this concept can help greatly in understanding the sign and configuration of the ST-T complex and in differentiating between primary and secondary repolarization abnormalities (see below).[14,45-49,449]

Whatever other factors may be at work, the process of repolarization is influenced by the route of depolarization.[48,50] If the ventricles are depolarized by some pathway other than the normal one, repolarization cannot be expected to follow its usual route; thus, change in the form of ST-T can be interpreted only as it relates to the associated QRS. If a heart with perfectly normal metabolic and physiologic processes has some small anatomic lesion that interferes with electrical conductivity of the left branch of the bundle of His, an old scar perhaps, the left ventricle is depolarized by a route other than normal, and the QRS is modified accordingly. This lesion does not influence the physiology of repolarization but does change its course so that the curve reflecting it is different from what it would be in the absence of the lesion. This is a *"secondary" T-wave abnormality*, i.e., it is entirely a consequence of the QRS change and does not indicate any physiologic or metabolic dysfunction of the myocardium. It is not really a functional abnormality at all but a statistical one related to form. Similarly, a heart with a normal QRS may be influenced by some drug or disease that does not cause structural change but does modify repolarization so that the ST-T complex is altered: a *"primary" T-wave abnormality*. It is possible, of course, for both primary and secondary T-wave abnormalities to be present at the same time, but study of the ventricular gradient is necessary to evaluate this hypothesis.

An analogy has been suggested to illustrate the difference between primary and secondary T-wave changes. The ST-T complex may be compared to the course taken by a water skier, while the QRS complex is represented by the motor boat. The skier need not follow exactly in the wake of the boat but he certainly must follow it in any general sense of the word. If he criss-crosses the wake of a boat that takes a "normal" course across the lake, his track represents primary T-wave abnormality; if, on the other hand, he follows exactly behind the boat but the boat pursues an erratic course, his route corresponds to secondary T-wave abnormalities.

The relative instability of the repolarization complex is at once a great help and a great danger in clinical electrocardiography. If it were necessary for there to be QRS abnormalities in order for electrocardiographic diagnoses to be made, we should be limited for the most part to diagnosing things that have resulted in anatomic change in the myocardium or conduction system. The ST-T complex is influenced easily by many things, though, and it is findings in this area that one is called upon most often to interpret. Remember that the only way a T wave can vary is in sign, amplitude, duration, or some combination of these, and that changes can be induced by many things from the drinking of cold water or changes in position to myocardial infarction or diphtheritic myocarditis. T-wave findings can serve often to support clinical diagnoses but only rarely can they establish a diagnosis themselves. They must be evaluated always in light of their associated QRSs and in their proper spatial orientation. The greatest danger to be avoided in electrocardiography in general is reading too much into findings, and this is especially true with the T wave.

The *U wave* should be mentioned for the sake of completeness.[51,52] It is a small deflection following T and identifiable in most tracings, especially in the right precordial leads. Its significance is poorly understood, and it merits attention only rarely. It probably is related in some way to ventricular repolarization.[431,670]

CHAPTER IV

Reference Frames

The reference frame in which events occur must be understood before those events can be analyzed appropriately. The structural and functional bases for the electrical events of the heartbeat have been considered, and now the framework in which their graphic representation is viewed must be identified. The figure with which we are concerned, the electrocardiogram, represents the net value of all electrical forces in a series of instants plotted against time on several projections, or leads, that are oriented so as to display this value in three dimensions. A discription of these leads has been chosen as the starting point for discussion of electrocardiography. A well-known poem by John Godfrey Saxe based on an ancient and even better known fable concerning the importance of reference frames provides an analogy.

THE BLIND MEN AND THE ELEPHANT

It was six men of Indostan
To learning much inclined,
Who went to see the Elephant
(Though all of them were blind),
That each by observation
Might satisfy his mind.

The First approached the Elephant,
And happening to fall
Against his broad and sturdy side,
At once began to bawl:
"God bless me! But the Elephant
Is very like a wall!"

The Second, feeling of the tusk,
   Cried, "Ho! What have we here
So very round and smooth and sharp?
   To me 'tis mighty clear
This wonder of an Elephant
   Is very like a spear!"

The Third approached the animal,
   And happening to take
The squirming trunk within his hands,
   Thus boldly up and spake:
"I see," quoth he, "the Elephant
   Is very like a snake!"

The Fourth reached out an eager hand,
   And felt about the knee.
"What most this beast is like
   Is mighty plain," quoth he;
"Tis clear enough the Elephant
   Is very like a tree!"

The Fifth who chanced to touch the ear
   said: "E'en the blindest man
Can tell what this resembles most;
   Deny the fact who can,
This marvel of an Elephant
   Is very like a fan!"

The Sixth no sooner had begun
   About the beast to grope,
Then, seizing on the swinging tail
   That fell within his scope,
"I see," quoth he, "the Elephant
   Is very like a rope!"

And so these men of Indostan
   Disputed loud and long,
Each in his own opinion
   Exceeding stiff and strong,
Though each was partly in the right,
   And all were in the wrong!

The Moral:
So oft in theologic wars,
The disputants, I ween,
Rail on in utter ignorance
Of what each other mean,
And prat about an Elephant
Not one of them has seen!

This can be interpreted as a statement of the problem at hand. Assume that we do not know what an elephant looks like but that we have one before us completely enclosed in a big box. An obvious way to find out what he looks like is to bore holes in the box and look at him. Let us bore three holes and label them 1, 2, and 3 (Figure 4-1). We look through these and see a forehead, side, and tail in that order: 1, 2, 3, forehead, side, tail. This is described as a normal elephant. We go away for a while and then come back and find that through hole 1 we see a tail, through hole 2 a side, and through hole 3 a forehead. On purely empirical grounds the elephant must now be classified as abnormal because the picture is different from that just defined as normal. This is illogical, of course, since it is clear to us that he has just turned around in the box. If we were to look in holes 1, 2, and 3, though, and see a forehead, tail, and side, then we should know there really was something wrong with the elephant. This is evident only because, contrary to the initial assumption, we do know what an elephant looks like. We are not impressed by the relation of its parts to the box but recognize it at once when those parts bear an abnormal relationship to each other.

Now the analogy should be obvious. The box is the body, the elephant represents the electrophysiology of the heart (the unknown), the holes are the leads, and the view we get through the holes is the electrocardiogram itself. Just as we can punch as many holes in the box as necessary to get a really good view of the elephant from all directions, so we can make as many leads from as many points on the surface of the body as necessary to get a good view of the anatomy and electrical activity of the heart, at least to the extent that the electrocardiogram can be interpreted as a reflection of these. As a matter of fact, it is appropriate to think of leads as views in which one looks from the positive electrode toward the negative one. And, by the same token that we know what a normal elephant looks like and are not likely to be fooled into thinking he is abnormal

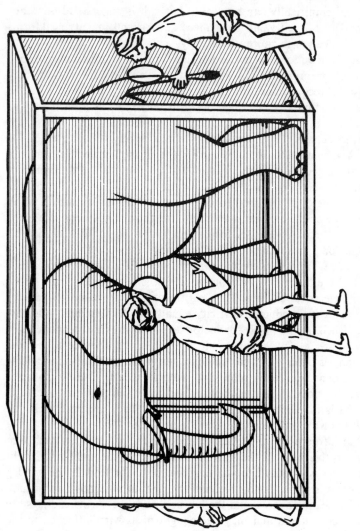

Figure 4-1. An elephant in a box.

simply because he has turned around in the box, it is possible to develop a concept of the duration, orientation, contour, and interrelation of the several components of the spatial electrocardiogram that will help in evaluating their normality or abnormality. Patterns learned empirically can be useful, but if it is understood how they were derived their value is enhanced and variants and atypical forms can be dealt with more confidently.

In order for electrocardiograms to be comparable to one another, in order for any conclusion to be drawn from them, they must be recorded according to a set of rules, and these must be understood by all concerned; the electrodes must be attached to the body so as to provide a standard reference frame; Professor Einthoven was the one who devised the system still in use.

A galvanometer is an instrument for measuring electricity and an electrocardiograph is a galvanometer set up to record difference of potential between two points, voltage; when one pole of the galvanometer is attached to one part of the body by means of an electrode and the other to another part, the arrangement is referred to as a lead. As a basis for establishing a standard lead system, Professor Einthoven identified a series of assumptions, or hypotheses, regarding the electrical properties of the body. He observed that 1) the heart may be thought of as a single dipole, a pair of opposite electrical charges; 2) it is at the center of a volume conductor (a mass that conducts electricity equally in all directions — as distinguished from a linear conductor such as a wire) the components of which are all of equal conductivity; 3) the shoulders and the symphysis pubis are in the same frontal plane with the heart, and 4) equidistant from each other and from the heart. These hypotheses have withstood the test of the time and study and continue to serve as the basis for clinical electrocardiography. They are implicit in the well-known Einthoven triangle (Figure 4-2A). To record lead 1, the left arm (representing the left shoulder in the triangle) is attached to the positive pole of the galvanometer, while the right arm (right shoulder) is attached to the negative pole; for lead 2, the left leg (symphysis pubis) is positive, and the right arm negative; for lead 3, the left leg is positive, and the left arm negative. Arms and legs are linear conductors and may be thought of as wires attached to the apices of the triangle.

Findings in one frontal plane lead may be related to those in others by superimposing them on this triangle, and the figure known as the triaxial reference system (Figure 4-2B) simplifies this procedure. Here the leads are represented as having a common zero point in the center while retaining the same polarity and angular relationship to each other that obtains in the triangle. It is easy to draw lines representing forces on this figure; the center is already defined and only one point needs to be identified from the tracing.

Einthoven's original three leads still are used and are still sometimes called "standard" or "bipolar" leads despite the fact that a standard tracing now utilizes 12 leads, and the nature of a galvanometer makes it necessary for any lead to have two poles. To call leads 1, 2, and 3 bipolar with the implication that the others are not is incorrect but probably does serve some purpose. Early in the development of electrocardiography it was suspected that useful information might be obtained if variations in potential at a point could be measured with reference to another point at which the potential remained stable. Such a system would provide effectively "unipolar" leads, since the change reflected would be taking place at only one point; the V leads approach this ideal very closely.

While one cannot place an electrode at the center of the volume conductor represented by the body, Wilson and co-workers[32] showed that it is possible to construct a lead system that, assuming Einthoven's hypotheses to be true, can provide a point the electrical potential of which does not vary and which thus can be defined as zero. Potential variations at any point on the body can be measured against this, and for practical purposes one has a truly unipolar lead. This central terminal is called the Wilson terminal and leads made with it "V" leads (V stands for voltage). Its connections are shown in Figure 4-3. In essence the system is based on Kirchhoff's law, which says that the algebraic sum of the electrical potentials in a closed network of wires is zero. The value of a force as seen from any lead will vary with the direction of the force, but the sum of its values in all leads will remain constant and may be used as a point of reference for evaluating changes. The V leads also include a relatively large resistance in each lead so that variations in skin resistance are small by comparison and do not affect the tracing significantly.

The six standard positions for the exploring chest electrodes are located with reference to easily identifiable landmarks on the bony thorax.[30] Position one is in the fourth intercostal space just to the right of the sternum; two, fourth intercostal space just to the left of the sternum; three, halfway between two and four; four, fifth inter-

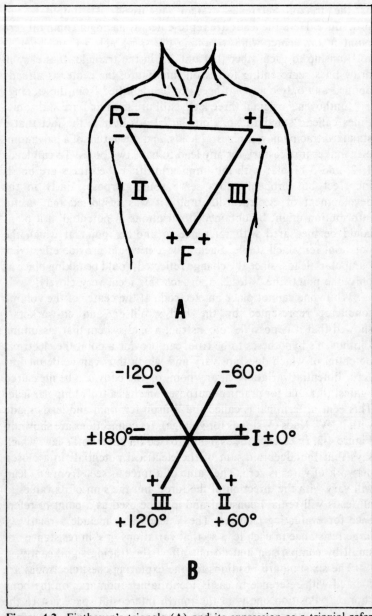

Figure 4-2. Einthoven's triangle (A) and its expression as a triaxial reference system (B).

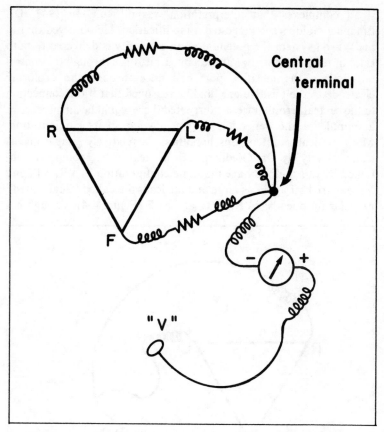

Figure 4-3. Wilson's central terminal of zero potential (V leads).

costal space in the left midclavicular line; five, the anterior axillary line at the same horizontal level as four; and six, the same level in the midaxillary line. When the precordial electrode is connected to the positive pole of the glavanometer, an upright deflection in one of these leads means that the net electrical force in the myocardium at that moment is directed toward it.

The six precordial V leads have been accepted as standard since shortly after their introduction, but the application of the unipolar concept to the frontal plane, leads VR, VL, and VF, resulted in such small complexes that interpretation was difficult. In 1942, Dr. Emanuel Goldberger suggested a modification. He observed that in the Wilson system the potential at an extremity is delivered to both sides of the galvanometer at the same time, once through the central terminal to the negative pole and once through the exploring electrode to the positive one, and he reasoned that if the connection to the central terminal were interrupted there would be an increase in amplitude of the deflection with no change in its configuration. Mathematical proof of this hypothesis is relatively simple and is stated clearly by Dr. Goldberger in his text.[31] The complexes obtained by this method have the same configuration as VR, VL, and VF but are half again as large and the leads are called "augmented" unipolar limb leads: aVR, aVL, and aVF (Figure 4-4). Though not

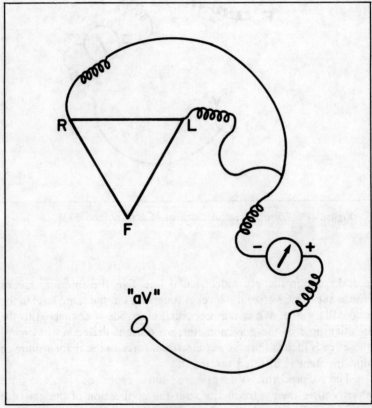

Figure 4-4. Goldberger's terminal, "augmented unipolar leads" (aV).

truly unipolar at all, of course, they have been accepted in principle, and aVR, aVL, and aVF are now standard. They fit easily into the Einthoven triangle to make a hexaxial reference system with 30° between each pair of lead lines (Figure 4-5). When questions of amplitude are involved, it must be remembered that the augmented unipolar limb leads do not produce exactly the same deflection of the stylus for a given voltage change as do the original three leads and this must be compensated for in constructing figures.

The technique for recording electrocardiograms that is now standard provides six leads in the frontal plane and six in the horizontal; the unknown is a three-dimensional phenomenon, and the EKG expresses it that way.

Orthogonal Reference Frames

It is universal practice to express the concept of space in terms of

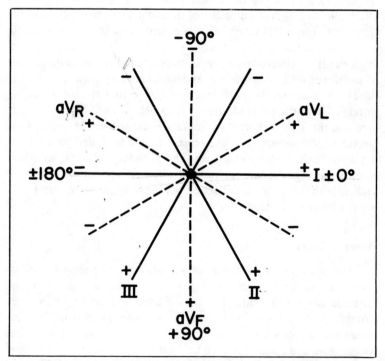

Figure 4-5. The hexaxial reference system for the frontal plane.

height, width, and depth, or lateral, vertical, and posteroanterior dimensions, defining an *orthogonal reference system*,[59] one in which the three dimensions are perpendicular to each other. In electrocardiographic terminology such a reference figure consists of X (horizontal), Y (vertical), and Z (posteroanterior) leads. Einthoven's hypotheses provide satisfactory X and Y information in leads 1 and aVF; no satisfactory Z lead has been derived yet, but it can be approximated usefully by V_1. Much effort has been spent in research aimed at devising a truly orthogonal lead system corrected for variations in the electrical characteristics of the body,[19,21] but none has been accepted generally.

Vector Analysis

From here on it will be helpful to use the word *vector*. In the context of the present subject a vector is a line used to represent a force. It is defined as having three characteristics, magnitude, sense, and direction; its length is a measure of the strength, or magnitude, of the force (voltage in this case); it has a positive end and a negative end; and it is pointed in some direction (up, down, right, left, forward, backward). In electrocardiography accurate indication of magnitude is usually of little consequence, and we do not pay much attention to it. This means that the exact length of the vectors in the examples is rarely of importance; traditionally the QRS is represented by a long one and the T by a short one. Sense is indicated by the angle of the vector with reference to a line representing a lead, and direction by an arrowhead to show which way the boundary of potential difference is moving. When a vector points toward a positive electrode, it indicates that a positive deflection will be written in the lead represented by that electrode.

Mean Vectors

The projection of a force, or vector, on a line must be understood. Consider a force starting at the center of the heart and directed toward the patient's left shoulder (Figure 4-6A). As seen from lead aVL, this would appear as a positive quantity of the same magnitude as the vector itself because the vector is parallel to the line of that lead and pointed toward its positive electrode. Seen from lead 1, the value still would be positive but not so great as in aVL, and

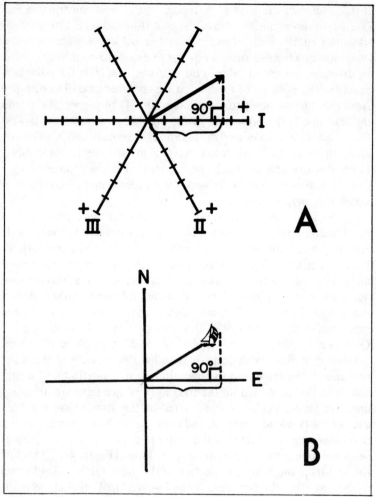

Figure 4-6. Projection of a vector.

there would be no projection at all on lead 2 as the force is perpendicular to that line. The projection on lead 3 would be negative. This is strictly analogous to the problem in high school geometry books in which one is required to figure how far to the east a boat has traveled after a given time during which it is moving, say, northeast (Figure 4-6B). One draws an east-west line (lead I), chooses a starting point on it (the center of the triaxial reference figure), and constructs a line (vector) to represent the path of the boat (force), taking into account its northeasterly course (direction and sense) and distance covered (magnitude). One determines how far due east the boat has traveled by dropping a perpendicular to the east-west line from the point representing the position of the boat at the specified time. The distance from the starting point to the intersection of the perpendicular and the lead line is the projection of the boat's course on the east-west line, a measure of its easterly progress. If the course had been directly north or south, there would have been no easterly component. From this example it should be apparent that *the projection of a force is maximal on a line to which it is parallel and zero on one to which it is perpendicular.*

Depolarization of the ventricular walls can be represented as many vectors pointing outward from the cavities in all directions. It requires about 0.06 to 0.08 sec for the whole mass to be depolarized. Forces in effect at a given instant during this time may be averaged and expressed as a single "instantaneous" vector, but at this stage of our discussion, it is convenient to think of all forces generated during the whole process as summed and expressed as a single vector representing the whole QRS. This may be derived by observing the QRS as recorded in any two leads, say 1 and 3. In each lead, the area subtended by positive deflections is added algebraically to the negative area in the same lead to determine the mean deflection for that lead, and this is plotted on the triaxial reference figure in arbitrary units. A perpendicular is constructed at the appropriate point on each of the two leads selected, and these perpendiculars intersect at a point that when connected to the center of the figure by a line, represents the summation of the two original forces (Figure 4-7). This line (or vector) is the frontal projection of the mean QRS and is known as the "axis" of the complex. It can be calculated precisely in millivolt-seconds, but this would require tedious measurement and is not practical or even useful for clinical purposes; it can be recognized easily by inspection. The lead in which the net QRS area is most nearly zero is the lead to which the force it represents is most nearly perpendicular, and its direction is determined by its projection on other leads. For instance, if the net QRS area is approximately zero in lead 3, the axis is either $+30°$ or $-150°$. If in the same tracing the net value of QRS in lead 1 is positive, then the axis is at $+30°$; if negative, $-150°$. The validity of this can be demonstrated by observing the QRS in other leads; with the axis at +30° the mean value in lead 1 must equal that in lead 2, since they are equidistant from the force indicated. A byproduct of this approach is renewed confidence in the dependability of Einthoven's premises. This technique of estimating frontal QRS orientation is accurate to about ±15°.[53,54] It is a common practice to determine the axis on the basis of the amplitude of the QRS deflections alone, not taking into account the duration. This results in figures that correlate positively with those based on area, but to express the value any closer than about 15° can lead to a false sense of security by giving the illusion of accuracy greater than the method affords.[53,416]

By dropping a perpendicular from the end of the axis vector to any lead, the mean deflection of the QRS in that lead will be indicated, confirming the observation that information contained in any lead may be obtained from any two other leads in that plane

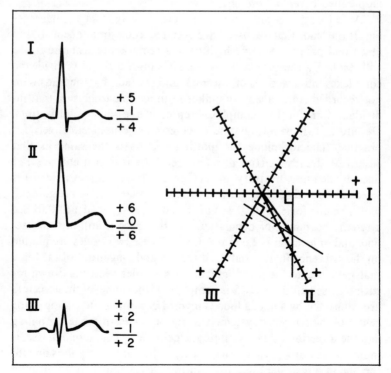

Figure 4-7. Derivation of mean frontal QRS (the axis).

whose relationship to each other is known. Since this is true, one may reasonably ask why it is that we routinely make six leads in the frontal plane instead of only two. The answer is that it is easier to let the machine write all these views than to have to construct them. In terms of the elephant in the box, it is easier to bore several holes to get a better view than it is to draw on one's knowledge of the anatomy of the elephant and interpolate what must lie between what can be seen through two holes.

The Vectorcardiogram

In discussing axis and vectors, the QRS has been considered only as a mean, but it can be studied in more detail by thinking of it as a continuum of events that can be plotted as a series of *instantaneous vectors*. The figure formed by connecting the ends of all these is a loop called a *vectorcardiogram*.

A vectorcardiogram can be constructed easily from a scalar tracing. If the leads that are used have been recorded simultaneously and at a rapid paper speed and high gain, a remarkably accurate figure will result; if a routine tracing is used, it is more difficult to divide the complexes into fractions of a second, and the fact that the leads were not recorded simultaneously makes it impossible to be sure that individual points in two complexes represent the same point in time. Despite this, however, routine tracings can be used effectively for practice. The technique for plotting vectors is the same as that described already. A triaxial reference figure is drawn and the lead lines divided into arbitrary units (Figure 4-8). A complex in lead 1 is selected for analysis and one in lead 3. Let us say that we are going to plot a vector for each 0.01 sec of the complex. In lead 1 at 0.01 sec after the beginning of depolarization, the trace is still at the baseline, and in lead 3 it is 2.0 mm below it. These two values are plotted on the reference figure, and the direction and magnitude of the force that gave rise to them are indicated. A similar vector is drawn for each 0.01 sec until the QRS is complete. If the points of these vectors are connected by a line, a loop is formed beginning and ending at the center of the reference system. This figure is known as the QRS loop and the direction of its inscription, clockwise or counterclockwise, is indicated. By dropping a series of perpendiculars from points on it to the line of a lead the exact form of the QRS complex in any lead in the frontal plane may be derived, demonstrating again that all of the

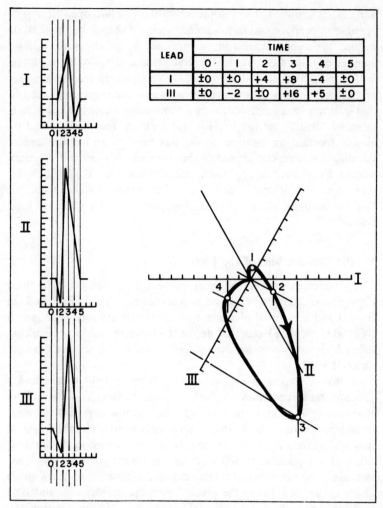

LEAD	TIME					
	0	1	2	3	4	5
I	±0	±0	+4	+8	−4	±0
III	±0	−2	±0	+16	+5	±0

Figure 4-8. Construction of the QRS loop in the frontal plane, relationship of scalarcardiogram and vectorcardiogram.

information in a given plane is contained in the wave forms of any two leads in that plane. This same technique may be extended, of course, to derive the P wave and the ST-T-U. As long ago as the early 1920s, QRS loops, called monocardiograms, were derived from frontal leads,[55] but instruments that could display such a figure were not available until the development of the oscilloscope. Now it is possible to produce two simultaneous views of the varying potentials within the myocardium and to indicate the result as an infinite number of instantaneous vectors describing a series of loops just as in the one constructed above, a VCG. Vectorcardiography has theoretical advantages over conventional scalar electrocardiography in that information is represented as a continuous whole instead of as a series of "stills," but the VCG is still a net, or mean, value and its most important application so far has been as an aid for understanding the interrelationship of the parts of the more useful scalar tracing. Problems limiting its clinical usefulness are the difficulty in evaluating time intervals, and thus disturbances of mechanism, the still cumbersome means of recording, and lack of a standard lead system.[55,56]

Spatial Relationships of the EKG

In order to picture the electrical events of the heart in three dimensions, their projection on two planes must be studied, and the frontal and horizontal planes are the ones that are used. The lateral (X) and vertical (Y) axes that define the frontal plane have been considered already; now we are ready to add the Z axis, a postero-anterior one.

Consider a pair of scissors held between a light source and a groundglass screen upon which they cast a shadow. You are looking from the other side of the screen at this shadow and wish to determine what relation the blades of scissors bear to each other, that is, how widely they are open. If the scissors are held perfectly horizontal, it is not possible to tell whether the blades are open or closed because their shadows are superimposed. In order to learn more about the angle between the blades, then, the scissors are rotated so that they are vertical, i.e., parallel to the screen. In this position, the angle between the blades is clear from the projection. If the scissors could not be rotated with relation to the screen, it would be equally effective to rotate the screen and the light source around the scissors.

This situation is comparable to the electrocardiographic problem of determining the spatial relation between the QRS and T vectors; the heart cannot be moved, but it can be observed from other views. The projection on the frontal plane has been discussed already. The posteroanterior projection is studied in the horizontal plane represented by precordial leads, and these two planes, perpendicular to each other, represent space.

At this point a reference figure must be introduced for the horizontal plane (Figure 4-9). This figure is a circle with precordial leads indicated on it. While of more recent origin than the triaxial system used for frontal leads, not so standard, and much less accurate, it suffices for an introduction to spatial orientation of electrical forces and is helpful in many clinical situations.[57,58] The center of this circle is the same point in space as the center of the triaxial reference system, and its circumference represents an arbitrary boundary of the volume conductor that is the torso. A line extending from the center to a point midway between the V_1 and V_2 electrode positions, and one from the center to the V_6 position, define an angle of 90°, and the angle between each two consecutive precordial leads may be considered as 20°. The projection of forces on this figure is determined from appropriate leads in exactly the same manner as in the frontal plane. Here, though, simple inspection is an even more easily applicable technique than before, especially when mean vectors are being considered.

Consider once again a muscle strip in a volume conductor observed in the plane of the paper as in earlier examples (Figure 4-10A). A unipolar electrode observing the process of depolarization from the end of the strip toward which the boundary of potential difference is moving will record a completely positive deflection; one at the opposite end, a completely negative one; and an electrode at the center of the strip will write a positive deflection during the first half of depolarization while the process is approaching it, and a negative one of exactly the same dimensions during the last half because the process is now receding from it and it faces the negative side of the boundary of potential difference. Similarly, exploring electrodes positioned closer to the origin of the impulse than to its termination will write predominantly negative deflections and those closer to the other end of the strip predominantly positive ones. The farther these exploring electrodes are placed from the strip the smaller the deflection will be (law of inverse squares), but the configuration of the curves will remain the same. The curve recorded from any electrode equidistant from the ends of the strip will be equiphasic plus-minus — a "transitional" curve. Thus, one can define a plane perpendicular to the line (vector) representing depolarization and equidistant from its ends; a transitional curve can be recorded from any point on this plane (Figure 4-10B). Because the algebraic sum of the deflections of a transitional curve is zero, this plane is called a "tran-

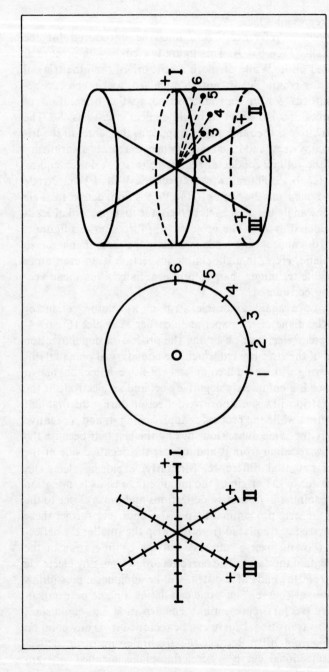

Figure 4-9. Spatial reference figures. The frontal system on the left is the triaxial expression of Einthoven's triangle; the horizontal one in the center is arbitrary and shows the precordial lead positions as viewed from above and separated by 20°; the drawing at the right shows the two figures superimposed. (A device representing these figures and useful in developing spatial concepts of the electrocardiogram can be obtained from: Medical Plastics, 421 Avery Street, Decatur, Georgia, 30038).

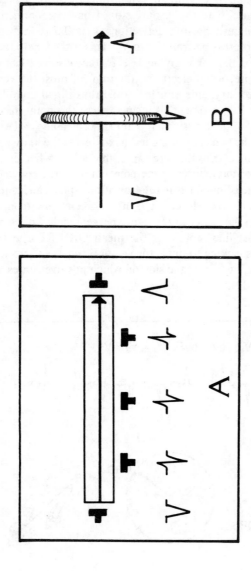

Figure 4-10. Relationship of forces to tracing. A represents a muscle strip observed by a series of electrodes, each representing the positive pole of a lead. As depolarization advances from left to right, an upstroke is written from electrodes ahead of the boundary of potential difference and a negative one from those behind it, with an equiphasic curve being recorded at the center of the system. The same information is presented in slightly different form in B; the tracing recorded from any point on a plane equidistant from the ends of the force and perpendicular to it will be equiphasic, the null, or transitional, plane.

sitional" or "null" plane, another example of the fact that the projection of a force on a plane to which it is perpendicular is zero.

In the illustration, one familiar with the precordial electrocardiogram will note that the progression from predominantly negative to predominantly positive deflections is similar to that seen in the usual QRS progression from V_1 to V_6. This is the key to location in this plane of the force giving rise to the observed curves. Somewhere in the precordial electrocardiogram (of most subjects), interpolating if necessary, one can locate a transitional complex, usually at about the V_4 position. This means that at this point the exploring electrode is on the transitional plane described above, i.e., it is equidistant from the two ends of the unknown force. We know that this plane is perpendicular to the force at its midpoint. A line drawn between the center of the figure and the point on its periphery where the transitional curve is found lies in the transitional plane and is perpendicular to the unknown force. It is no problem now to draw another line through the center of the figure perpendicular to the one just drawn. This last line represents the mean QRS force in this plane, and all that is lacking to finish the vector is to put an arrow on the proper end to point toward the side on which positive curves are recorded (Figure 4-11).

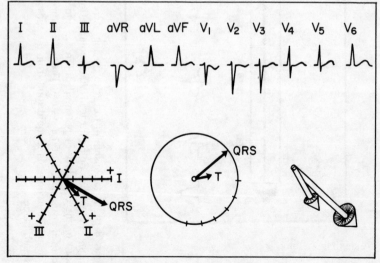

Figure 4-11. Mean spatial QRS and T.

The spatial orientation of the vector now has been fixed; we know which way it points laterally, vertically, and posteroanteriorly. To express this accurately in a diagram requires two figures, of course, but the PA direction can be suggested effectively by adding a shaded arrowhead to the vector drawn in the plane of the paper. The T vector is plotted in the same manner, and the spatial relation between the two becomes clear. Practice helps a great deal, and it does not take much for the method to become second nature — for one to think of the forces in their spatial orientation without even realizing it. It is possible to construct spatial loops, but it is not often that such a relatively laborious procedure adds much to the interpretation of the tracing.*

Derivation of mean vectors from electrocardiograms should be recognized from the beginning as a method intended to inculcate in the student early in the course of his study a concept of the spatial orientation of forces and their interrelationships, to prevent his thinking of individual electrocardiographic leads as separate things. There is some danger, however, of making this same mistake with regard to the vectors themselves, of coming to think of them as things and to expect them to interpret electrocardiograms.[284] Vectors are a means of expressing concepts; they do not "cause" anything.

Remember: 1) A lead should be thought of as a view of the electrophysiology of the heart with the viewer looking from the positive electrode toward the center of the heart. 2) All leads view the whole process of depolarization and repolarization as if the whole heart were equally remote from the exploring electrode. 3) No lead is better than any other except as its view of the event in question is more effective. 4) It is necessary to look at the whole picture from all points of view in order to see what is going on and to do this the observer must have an understanding of the reference frame with which he is working.

---

*A small model that is effective as an aid in visualizing the three-dimensional nature of electrocardiography is available from: Medical Plastics, 421 Avery Street, Decatur, Georgia 30038.

CHAPTER V

The Normal Electrocardiogram

Now that the anatomic and physiologic bases of electrocardiography — the rules of the game — and how they fit into the big picture of clinical medicine have been presented, it is time to examine the tracing itself, to identify its components and to name them (Figures 5-1 and 5-2).

The rectilinear coordinates on which the tracing is described are one millimeter apart with every fifth line accentuated. When the paper is drawn past the stylus at exactly 25 mm per second, the time between two vertical lines (the little squares) is 0.04 sec and that between two heavy lines (the big squares) is 0.20 sec. Standard calibration is such that one millivolt produces a deflection of 10 millimeters. The vertical lines in the margin of the chart are three seconds apart.

The baseline, the level to which everything is referred, is the flat line recorded when there is no difference of potential in the system. Ideally, the PQ segment, J point, T-U segment, and U-P segment are all at this same zero level. In practice, though, this is not often the case, and the PQ segment, or the point at which it joins the QRS complex, is arbitrarily taken as the level of the baseline. A *wave*, or *deflection*, is a complete round trip of the stylus from baseline to baseline; irregularities — notching and slurring — may occur on upstroke or downstroke, but the name does not change until the trace crosses the baseline. The first wave in the cardiac cycle is a small one produced by depolarization of the atria and called *P*. A normal P is small, may be positive, negative, or biphasic, and occurs before each ventricular complex. Atrial repolarization theoretically produces a deflection, the T_a or P_t, but in practice no such wave is visible, presumably because it is very small and obliterated by the QRS.

During passage of the impulse through the AV junction the trace remains isoelectric until depolarization of the ventricles begins. The

44

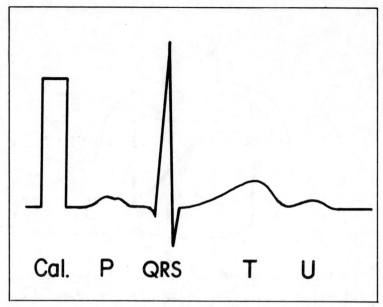

Figure 5-1. The waves of the electrocardiogram. A wave is defined as the curve written from the time the stylus leaves the baseline until it returns to it, including both initial and terminal limbs and often notched; the name does not change until the trace crosses the baseline. The calibration (cal) is the curve written by exactly one millivolt; amplitudes are always expressed to a base of one millivolt equals one centimeter.

time between the beginning of the P wave and that of the QRS is called the *PR interval* (though it may really be a PQ).

The *QRS complex* is the electrocardiographic manifestation of depolarization of the ventricles and this generic name applies no matter what the individual components. A *Q wave* is a negative deflection that initiates the complex and is followed by a positive wave; an *R wave*, any positive deflection; and an *S wave* is a negative deflection following a positive one. Note that there are two names for negative deflections and that distinction between them depends on their relation to a positive one; if there is no positive deflection the completely negative complex is a *QS*. When there is more than one positive or negative deflection, those following the first may be designated by "prime" marks (RSR', QRSR'S'); relative values may be

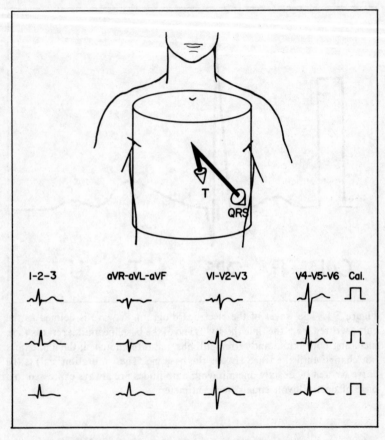

Figure 5-2. The normal electrocardiogram.

indicated by use of upper and lower case letters (qR, qRs, Qr). During repolarization of the ventricles, a relatively slow, smooth deflection, the *T wave*, is written. The terminology of this curve is confusing because the name T is used for the whole thing as well as for its terminal portion selectively and is the same whether the deflection is positive or negative. The proximal part is called the *ST* segment. The term *ST-T complex* emphasizes that the whole curve is meant when use of T alone might leave uncertainty. The last wave in the cycle is much smaller and less clearly defined than the others — the *U wave*.

Mechanism

The mechanism is a statement of the rate, rhythm, and locus or the pacemaker for the atria, that for the ventricles, and the relationship between them. Analysis of the mechanism is a part of the description of every tracing. In the normal heart the impulse arises in the sinus node and traverses the atria, AV junctional tissue, and ventricles, producing the P, QRS, T, and U, in that order. There is no interference with conduction anywhere, and no ectopic pacemaker complicates the picture. This is a sinus mechanism. It is recognized by the one-to-one relation of atrial and ventricular complexes at a rate that may be anywhere between about 40 and 200 per minute but is usually between 50 and 100. The rhythm may vary a little but is very nearly regular, and the PR interval is no longer than 0.20 sec when the rate is less than 100.

Atrial Depolarization

The P wave reflects depolarization of the atria. It has two components: the first, derived from the right atrium, is directed downward, leftward, and a little anteriorly; and the second, representing the left, is directed downward, leftward, and posteriorly. Overall, the two curves present as a single wave, often slightly notched, directed downward and to the left, and usually with a small initial component directed anteriorly and a terminal one directed posteriorly. In the 12-lead tracing, P is usually positive in leads 1, 2, and V6, and biphasic (initially positive and terminally negative) in V1. It is often so small that identification is difficult, and it rarely exceeds 2 or 3 mm in amplitude and 0.10 sec in duration.

Ventricular Depolarization

The QRS is analyzed in terms of its duration, amplitude, contour, and orientation. In adults, the *duration* is about 0.06 to 0.08 sec with 0.10 sec as the upper limit of normal.[61] The maximal *amplitude* in lead 1, 2, or 3 (measured from the top of the R wave to the bottom of the S) is at least 0.5 mv, and the sum of SV_1 and RV_5 (or RV_6, whichever is taller) does not exceed 3.5 mv. Its *contour* may include any combination of positive and negative deflections depending upon the lead and the specific tracing concerned. All deflections are smooth and clean. Its *orientation* (axis) is to the left, downward, and dorsad, i.e., between about −30° and +90° in the frontal plane, and predominantly negative in V₁ progressing smoothly to predominantly positive in V₆.

Repolarization

Atrial repolarization would be represented by T_a or P_t, but no such wave is identifiable in the surface tracing of the normal individual.[395] The repolarization complex of the *ventricles,* the ST-T-U, like the QRS, has duration, amplitude, contour, and orientation, but absolute numbers for these are not so easy to specify. *Duration* is measured as the QT interval, electrical systole, and is usually about 0.40 sec. The *amplitude* of the T is judged by comparison to the QRS rather than by absolute standards. In leads in which the QRS is almost completely positive and the T is of the same sign, the amplitude of the T normally would be at least about 10% of that of the QRS. The normal ST-T *contour* can be described as departing from the baseline at an increasingly rapid rate until a maximum deflection is reached (the peak of the T) near its end, and a quick return to the baseline. The spatial *orientation* is judged in relation to the QRS rather than to the body and is normal when the angle between the QRS and T is small, not more than about 45° in the frontal plane or 60° in the horizontal.[14,63-65]

The *U wave* is identifiable in most normals as a small deflection following the T and usually is of the same sign as the T.

The *J point* is the point of juncture of the QRS and ST-T.

CHAPTER VI

Impulse Formation and Conduction

ANALYSIS

Introduction

The vocabulary that has evolved to describe disorders of cardiac mechanism is neither consistent nor logical and makes it difficult to say clearly just what one means. As understanding of the subject has grown, some words and names that seemed appropriate when first used have become less so, and the problem is made worse by the tradition for medical students to learn this clinical cant along with the fundamentals of physiology and anatomy. It is possible, though, to analyze findings in considerable detail and to untangle the terminology so that the jargon that doctors use — the words through which thought processes must pass on their way to being translated into patient care — can have meaning. Efforts have been made to lessen this problem by standardizing definitions,[556] but they are not likely to have much effect.

No classification of these disorders of impulse formation and conduction is altogether satisfactory, and in no other aspect of electrocardiography is its ultimately clinical, empirical nature quite so clear. Study of the cardiac mechanism means study of two subjects, impulse formation and impulse conduction. They must be analyzed separately, but to consider either as if it were completely distinct from the other would be inappropriate; they are too closely related. A few definitions and rules summarizing the anatomic and physiologic considerations discussed in Chapter III can serve as a starting point and provide guidelines.

1) The mechanism of the heartbeat is a statement, ultimately cast

in language that will be understood by the doctor who has to apply it, of the rate, rhythm, and locus of the pacemaker for the atria, the rate, rhythm, and locus of that for the ventricles, and the relationship between the two.

The word "rhythm," often used to imply all of this, obscures the problem; rhythm is a necessary word, used and understood by everyone, not just doctors, to indicate timing. Rhythm is an important feature of the heartbeat — but only one aspect of it, not the whole thing; "mechanism" leaves room for the other components.

The rate and rhythm of the atria and the ventricles can usually be determined objectively without difficulty, but naming the locus of the pacemaker for each and analyzing the relationship between events in the upper chambers and those in the lower require judgment. Consider: the atria and the ventricles are capable of beating independently, either consistently or intermittently, the impulse depolarizing either may originate in the other at a rapid rate or a slow one, the curves produced may be positive or negative, great or small, and only the net result of all this (as well as any other electrical activity in the body such as muscle tremor, the calibration signal, and various artifacts) is recorded. It is important to appreciate the difference between what can be demonstrated objectively and what is assumed to be the best explanation for it.

2) There are four places in the heart in which electrical impulses may arise (i.e., depolarization begins): the sinus node, the atria, the AV junction (a reasonably vague term that includes some atrial tissue, AV node, and His bundle), and the ventricles.

The first three of these are proximal to the bifurcation of the bundle of His and are referred to collectively as supraventricular. Any pacemaker other than the sinus node is ectopic by definition.

Electrical characteristics of cardiac cells may be described in terms of the time course of the voltage across their membranes, the difference between the value within the cell and a reference point outside it. The curves representing this transmembrane action potential vary among different types of cells and can be used to differentiate between those in which depolarization occurs spontaneously (automaticity) and those in which, for practical purposes, it does not. The first group are the pacemaker cells, and the latter are suited better for conduction. There is reason to believe that automaticity may, under some circumstances, be potential in any myocardial cell, but it is common only in the groups indicated above.[36,40,42,487]

3) The most rapidly firing pacemaker available to the atria drives them, and the same is true for the ventricles.

In the normal heart the rates inherent in the foci just named diminish in the order listed: sinus, 40-100; junction, about 50; and ventricles, about 30. If a higher, faster pacemaker fails to fire, the next one beneath it drives the ventricles, a *default*, or secondary, mechanism; if a lower pacemaker fires at a rate greater than that inherent in a higher one, it drives the chambers to which it is accessible, a *usurping*, or primary, mechanism.

4) The relationship between atrial and ventricular complexes, whether one is causally related to the other and in what manner, is almost completely a matter of interpretation.

Analysis of Atrial Activity

The atria may be electrically inactive, they may be depolarized in a regular, repetitive fashion, or their electrical activity may be grossly irregular with individual fibers acting on their own without coordination with the others.

1) *No activity.* The baseline is flat between ventricular complexes (there is no deflection between the U wave of one complex and the QRS of the next). This occurs when the atria are not beating at all or when there is a midjunctional pacemaker. In the latter case, the QRS rhythm is regular at a rate of somewhere around 50, and (presumably) the atria are depolarized at the same time as the ventricles so that P waves simply cannot be seen. Other explanations for absence of atrial activity include SA block — the impulse being formed in the sinus node but kept from entering the atria so that the atria are not depolarized. It has been proposed also that an impulse may reach the AV node from the sinus node by way of internodal pathways without depolarizing the atria, sinoventricular conduc-

tion.[484,491,498,519] It may be that atrial activity is present, but the complexes it produces are just too small to see.[485,498]

2) *Rate and rhythm.* In normal hearts, the atria are depolarized regularly, initiating each cardiac cycle and producing a deflection in the tracing, the P wave. In the normal heart, a P wave is a small deflection of low voltage and low frequency and (usually) regularly recurrent. It is a composite of two curves, the initial one written by depolarization of the right atrium to the left, downward, and anteriorly merging with that from the left atrium directed to the left, downward, and dorsad. The typical, normal P wave is positive in leads whose positive electrodes are left and/or down (1, 2, L, aVF, and/or 3). It usually has a small notch in frontal leads and is biphasic, initially positive and terminally negative, in V1.

Origin of an occasional P outside the sinus node is easy to recognize if most of the Ps are of sinus origin, because direct comparison is available and the ectopic one is different, but when all the Ps are alike it may not be possible on the basis of configuration alone to be sure where they originate. An impulse that arises low in an atrium proceeds in a direction approximately opposite to normal and produces a P that is clearly, and usually prominently, negative in 2, 3, and F, and, when identifiable, in lead I also. It often has a sharp "V" shape. Ps may or may not be followed by QRSs depending on their timing and the state of refractoriness of the tissues.

If there are no consistently identifiable P waves, and the baseline is not perfectly flat, then it follows that the atria must be fibrillating, since there is nothing else for them to do. But still the diagnosis of atrial fibrillation should be a positive one and not one of exclusion. Most of those in a position to be analyzing electrocardiograms have a pretty good idea of what atrial fibrillation is; they have seen the difference in the laboratory between rhythmic contraction of normal atria and the diffuse, uncoordinated, quivering activity of individual fibers in atrial fibrillation (when pronounced with a long i, the word sounds like what it means). In the electrocardiogram, the irregularly irregular undulation of the baseline characteristic of atrial fibrillation is easy to recognize at a glance, even for a beginner, when gross (as it often is) but the pattern, the coarseness/fineness, varies widely, and sometimes motion of the baseline is barely perceptible. It may be defined as present when the trace between no two consecutive pairs of ventricular complexes in the same lead look precisely the same. Remember that the whole tracing must be taken into account; bumps in the baseline that considered by themselves and in another context would be P waves may not be P waves here; significance, remember, is part of the definition. Differentiation between a P and a bump is often problematic. The ventricular rhythm in patients with atrial fibrillation is characteristically irregularly irregular, but this is not a criterion for the electrocardiographic diagnosis; when there is doubt, the regularity or irregularity of the ventricular response is helpful as an associated finding, but at this point, we are concerned only with electrocardiographic evidence of atrial activity.

3) *Locus of the atrial pacemaker*. Rate alone will not identify the origin of a P wave, but it is of help. In the adult human heart, the sinus node may function normally and effectively at rates varying from below 40 to perhaps 300 per minute. A useful figure to remember, though, is that in an adult having an electrocardiogram made at rest, the sinus rate rarely exceeds 140/min; when it does, there will be a clearly identifiable basis for it. This basis will not be apparent in the tracing, but the clinical setting must always be considered before a decision is reached. Increase in heart rate is the first response of the circulatory system to a demand for more oxygen, and the sinus rate frequently exceeds 140 and may reach 200 or more in patients who have such problems as infiltrative pulmonary disease, hyperpyrexia, hypermetabolic states, and/or shock.

P waves originating in the atria or AV junction may represent either usurpation of pacemaker activity at a rapid rate or response of a lower, slower pacemaker to failure of higher, faster ones to function, i.e., default. *Usurping* mechanisms are almost always at a rate of 160 or more, often between about 160 and 220 or very nearly exactly 300, but no absolutes can be stated. Most atria do not respond regularly at rates above 300; at this level they begin to fibrillate. *Default* mechanisms originating in the atria receive very little attention in the literature but do occur and fit perfectly logically in this system of classification. They are called high junctional, high nodal, low atrial, or left atrial mechanisms (all of which mean about the same thing). If the configuration of the P wave and the duration of the PR interval vary perceptibly within a given lead, a diagnosis of *"wandering atrial pacemaker"* may be made, but this is a term that has little clinical importance and probably should be considered a variant of normal.[36,504]

Analysis of Ventricular Activity

1) *Rate and rhythm*. In the normal heart the rate of the ventricles is equal to that of the atria, between about 50 and 100 per minute in most people. A *usurping* mechanism originating in the ventricles,

ventricular tachycardia, will almost always, but not always, be at a rate of 160 or greater but rarely over 200. The *default* rate for the ventricles, idioventricular mechanism, is below 40, usually very close to 30, and sometimes much slower. Ventricular *rhythm* should be evaluated as to its regularity or irregularity and its relation to atrial activity.

2) *Locus.* The first determination to be made is whether the pacemaker for the ventricles is above the bifurcation of the bundle of His, *supraventricular*, or below it, *ventricular*. There are two bases for this distinction, duration and rate, and neither is absolute. If the QRS is narrow (not wider than 0.10 sec by inspection), the implication is that the ventricles are depolarized over a normal route, that the impulse must have entered the ventricular conduction system above the bifurcation of the bundle of His. An obvious, and usually easily identifiable, exception is bundle branch block. If the ventricles are activated from a focus within their own substance (probably in the His-Purkinje system), the wave front spreads more slowly than normal and over an abnormal route and the QRS will be broader than normal and its configuration different from normal; "bizarre" is often used to describe it. Though of little consequence at this point, it is interesting to note that one can tell whether the impulse originates in the right ventricle or the left by the shape of the QRS; if in the left, the pattern is similar to right bundle branch block, and vice versa.

The other criterion is rate. Remember that the fastest functioning pacemaker available to the ventricles determines their rate. If there is no sinus or atrial activity, or if atrioventricular conduction is blocked completely, a distal focus must be called into play. The one with the inherent rate next below sinus is in the AV junction where the rate is of the order of 40-60; next, in the ventricles where the rate is about 30.

A problem arises when the rate is relatively rapid but the QRS is broad, and when the rate is slow but the QRS is narrow. The designation of a pacemaker in such instances is obviously arbitrary. From a clinical point of view the rate is the more important consideration, with faster default rates having a better prognosis than slower ones.

There are very few exceptions to the rule that anything that changes the configuration of the QRS complex represents structural change in the ventricular myocardium and/or its conduction system.

Quinidine and potassium toxicity can do it, though, and a tracing recorded at 50 mm per sec may simulate IV conduction abnormality. Unrecognized, any of these may be interpreted as evidence of ventricular origin of the QRS.

Relation Between Atria and Ventricles

In analyzing the relation between atrial and ventricular complexes, it must be recognized that whether ventricular depolarization is a consequence of atrial depolarization, whether there is a causal relation between P and QRS, is always and necessarily a matter of judgment; there is only one stylus, and it records on a single strip of paper the electrical activity of both atria and ventricles no matter what the functional relationship, if any, between the two may be. For instance, if there are both Ps and QRSs in a tracing, a PR interval, defined simply as the distance between the beginning of P and the beginning of QRS, can be measured even when there is complete AV block; when we say PR interval what we really mean is that we think the QRS complex following a P derived from the passage of the same impulse through the AV junction and into the ventricles, a matter of judgment — usually secure, but judgment nonetheless.

Relationship between atria and ventricles may be consistent or variable. If it is other than one-to-one, AV dissociation is said to be present; i.e., the atria and ventricles are disassociated, a-synchronous, and if it is complete there must be separate pacemakers for atria and ventricles. Dissociation may result from usurpation of ventricular pacemaker activity by a junctional focus so that the ventricles are refractory when the impulse from above reaches them, "interference dissociation," or to a discrepancy between the rate of input into the AV conduction system and its ability to conduct, AV block (see page 76).

Abnormalities of conduction pathways in the region of the AV node occur and may give rise to complex variations of mechanism (see page 68)

CHAPTER VII

Disorders of Impulse Formation

SUPRAVENTRICULAR MECHANISMS

Sinus Mechanism and Its Variants

The normal heartbeat is initiated by an impulse that arises in the sinus node, spreads over the atria, and then, after a pause, is delivered to the ventricles. The P wave records depolarization of the atria, the PR interval represents the interval between atrial and ventricular activity, and the QRS complex is written during depolarization of the ventricles. T represents ventricular repolarization. This sequence of events is called a *sinus mechanism*. There is one P for each QRS-T, and in the resting adult, the rate is between about 50 and 100 per minute; the rhythm is slightly irregular, usually cyclic with respiration, *sinus arrhythmia*. If the sinus node fails to initiate an impulse at the time expected but the next beat is a normal one, there is a longer interval than usual between two beats of sinus origin — a *sinus pause*. If sinus inactivity continues long enough, the next slower pacemaker will "escape" and produce a beat of junctional or ventricular origin. The ectopic focus in these instances commonly initiates only one beat, the sinus node promptly resuming its role as pacemaker.

Sinus tachycardia, a sinus mechanism at a rapid rate, is usually a normal response to a need for an increase in blood flow. The sinus node can initiate impulses up to a rate of over 200 per minute in healthy young people during vigorous exercise but rarely exceeds about 140 in hospitalized adults except in easily identifiable circumstances calling for an increase in blood flow, e.g., hyperpyrexia, thyrotoxicosis, pulmonary disease, shock, or acute blood loss. From the tracing alone, it is not always possible to differentiate between sinus tachycardia and atrial tachycardia, but it is rare for untreated atrial tachycardia to occur at a rate slower than about 160; rates between 140 and 160 often can be interpreted only with knowledge of the clinical picture; sinus rates in this range are more common than atrial.

In the perfectly normal individual with no impairment of cardiac structure or function, rates approaching 200 may be tolerated without ST-T abnormalities, but ST-T abnormalities that occur with tachycardia and are not present when the rate is slower may not be a cause for alarm or even for a diagnosis of heart disease.

Sinus bradycardia is characterized by nothing more than a slow rate, sometimes below 40 per minute. It is not unusual in healthy individuals, especially young athletes.

None of these variants is likely to be symptomatic or of clinical significance in itself. They are seen with particular frequency in children and in elderly people, especially those taking digitalis.

Sometimes a single complete cardiac cycle, a P-QRS-T, is missing while the regular rhythm continues. This is called *sino-atrial (SA) block*,[67,68,420,421,494,506] the inference being that an impulse occurred in the sinus node but did not enter the atria. The terminology of SA block is exceedingly complex and inconstant, and the hypotheses and assumptions that underlie the putative explanations of the findings are even more obscure than in most disorders of mechanism. The clinical importance of SA block is hard to evaluate because of difficulty in defining it precisely; it ranges from insignificant, merging with sinus arrhythmia and "wandering atrial pacemaker," to catastrophic when it is complete and no lower pacemaker takes over — literally cardiac standstill, an indication for insertion of an artificial ventricular pacemaker.[420,421] In some instances it may be provoked, or abolished, by quinidine.[651]

The concept of a *"wandering atrial pacemaker"*[36,627] is that some beats arise in the sinus node, some from sites in the atria, and some from the AV junction. It would be characterized by P waves whose configurations vary within a given lead and whose associated PR intervals shorten as the pacemaker approaches the AV junction. It is not a very important diagnosis and can be thought of as a variant of normal.

It has been proposed that the sinus pacemaker may function normally without producing any P waves at all — the impulse reaching the AV junction via preferential pathways of internodal conduction without depolarizing the atria, *sinoventricular conduction.*[491] This would produce a perfectly flat baseline between ventricular complexes and would be inseparable from the classic description of midjunctional mechanism.

The term *"sick sinus syndrome"* has been popularized to indicate a spectrum of clinical problems resulting from instability of the sinus node so that the rate varies between very slow and very fast and sometimes includes periods of asystole; it has been called "sluggish sinus" and "brady-tachy" syndrome also. The diagnosis is a clinical one, not an electrocardiographic one,[521,533] and other examples of sinus node dysfunction occur.[536,652-654]

Atrial dissociation has been reported.[74,424,476,479,524] *Intraatrial block* is rare but can be recognized in the electrocardiogram by an increased notching of P.[492]

Nature of Atrial Impulses

It is appropriate to understand as much as possible about the pathophysiology of disorders of electrical impulse formation, of course, but limitations of knowledge in this area are more apparent in planning treatment than in making an EKG diagnosis. That is, disorders can be identified and named from the electrocardiogram without knowing the means of their production. Identification of P waves and fibrillary waves, or of atrial inactivity, is usually not difficult (Figure 7-1).

For a long time it was taught that mechanisms of atrial origin were the result of "circus conduction" and students left medical school with the impression that this was established fact. Other possibilities had been considered, however, and in the early fifties Dr. Prinzmetal and his associates in California applied high speed movie techniques to study of the question.[69] Their observations sustained the view that atrial mechanisms are explained best in most instances by the presence of a single ectopic pacemaker. The matter is still debated,[70] and distinction between initiation of impulse formation in an atrial focus and the mechanism by which repetitive firing is sustained is an important one (see page 68).

Usurping Atrial Mechanisms

Premature atrial contractions (PACs) arise from foci in the atrial musculature. By definition, the P wave of a PAC is premature and, though it may not be clearly identifiable, its contour will be different

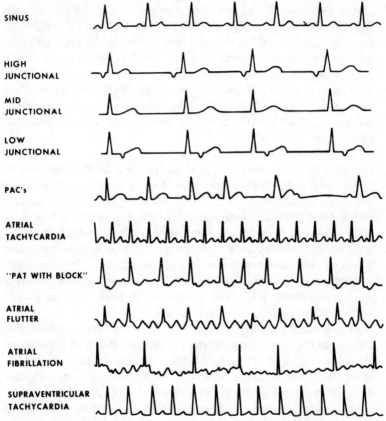

Figure 7-1. Supraventricular mechanisms. PACs = premature atrial contractions. The first PAC (fourth P-QRS-T) is conducted and the second one is blocked. "PAT with block" = paroxysmal atrial tachycardia with second degree AV block.

from normal. Its PR interval may be shorter than normal or, depending upon its timing with relation to the preceding beat and the refractory periods of the tissues involved, longer than normal;[423] it may be *blocked* completely so that a premature P wave occurs without a ventricular complex following it.[76] In most instances the QRS-T complex is normal because ventricular depolarization follows its usual course, but variations are common and related to refractoriness of the ventricular myocardium (see ventricular aberration, page 95). The pause following the PAC may or may not be compensatory, i.e., the interval between the beat preceding the PAC and that following it may be the same as if the PAC had not occurred. PACs may be frequent or rare, regular or irregular, unifocal or multifocal, isolated or in groups. If several appear together, there is a paroxysm of atrial tachycardia (PAT); if a PAC follows each sinus beat, there is *bigeminy* due to PAC, or atrial begeminy. *Atrial parasystole* occurs rarely (see page 75).

If the ectopic focus continues to fire, or its repetitive discharge is sustained by some other means, it usurps the role of pacemaker — *atrial tachycardia* (AT) (Figure 7-2). An important lead to recognition of atrial tachycardia is an atrial rate in excess of 160 per minute with normal QRS-T complexes each of which is preceded by a P. If no example of a P that is clearly of sinus origin is available for comparison, abnormality of P contour may not be recognizable, and differentiation on a purely electrocardiographic basis between sinus and atrial tachycardia is not possible. Atrial tachycardia is usually a *paroxysmal* event (PAT) and is common in healthy young people without other evidence of heart disease.

The literature on atrial *flutter* is confused by varying definitions; sometimes the term seems to refer to a disease and other times to an electrocardiographic pattern. All EKG definitions, though, include atrial complexes at a rapid rate (AT), with all ventricular complexes of supraventricular origin but at a slower rate (2° AV block) — i.e., atrial flutter has two components, atrial tachycardia and second degree AV block, and these can be identified separately. Second degree AV block in this setting does not imply impairment of AV conduction but simply that a disproportion exists between the rate at which impulses arrive at the AV junction and that at which they can be conducted, a physiologic or secondary block as distinguished from the pathologic, or primary, variety resulting from impairment of conduction. Electrocardiographically the result is the same in that there are more Ps than QRSs — all QRS complexes are derived from Ps but not all Ps are followed by QRSs (Figure 7-3).

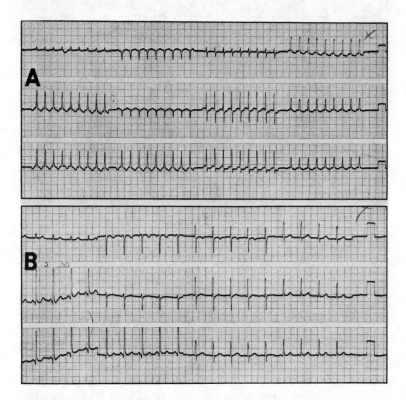

Figure 7-2. Supraventricular tachycardia. The upper tracing shows normal QRSs at a rate of 250 per minute but no discernible atrial activity. Low T voltage, wide QRS-T angle, and ST displacement probably mean coronary insufficiency, but at this rate this doesn't necessarily mean coronary artery disease. The lower tracing, from the same 18-year-old subject three hours later, is normal in all respects, and the sinus mechanism is clear and uncomplicated. All that can be said with confidence of the mechanism in the upper tracing is that it is of supraventricular origin with a rapid ventricular rate and a regular rhythm, i.e., supraventricular tachycardia. The probability is that the pacemaker is in the atria, and the findings support the clinical diagnosis of paroxysmal atrial tachycardia. In "PAT" atrial activity often is not clear, and the precise EKG diagnosis is supraventricular tachycardia. Other tachycardias of atrial origin — fibrillation and flutter — are often paroxysmal, too.

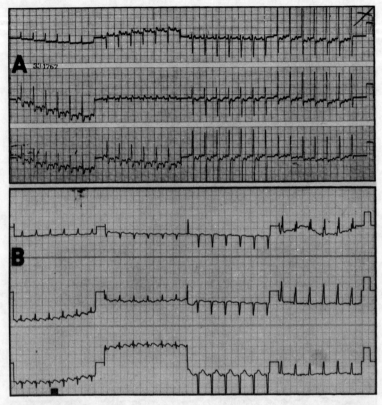

Figure 7-3. Atrial flutter. The atrial rate is about 300 in each tracing, and the ventricular rate 150. All ventricular complexes are of supraventricular origin, but not all supraventricular complexes (P waves or F waves) are followed by QRSs, i.e., second-degree AV block is present, and at this atrial rate it can be assumed to be a consequence of input into normal AV junctional tissue at a rate beyond that which can be conducted. This combination of events, atrial tachycardia and second-degree AV block, is called atrial flutter or, when the atrial rate is closer to 200 than 300, "PAT with block." Both tracings also show abnormally low T voltage, and in the lower one there is also an old anterior myocardial infarct.

A part of the traditional definition of atrial flutter is that there is continuous evidence of atrial activity, a serrated baseline with no flat space between P (or F) waves, and this is the basis for easy pattern recognition. In the typical case the atrial rate is very nearly exactly

300, there is two-to-one conduction, and the ventricular rate is 150 with a regular rhythm, but AV conduction may be inconstant so that the QRS rhythm is irregular. The key to the diagnosis is recognition of "the other P wave" and this may not be easy since it may be buried in a QRS or T.[83] It is usually seen best in leads 2, 3, aVF, and/or V1 as an unusual configuration of the early ST and is much easier to recognize if there is a previous tracing that shows a sinus mechanism. When suspected, carotid sinus pressure may be uncovered while a tracing is being made by increasing AV block and slowing the ventricular rate, or a PVC may have the same effect.

The rate of usurping atrial pacemakers varies widely, and impairment of AV conduction may range from minimal to complete. When the atrial rate is slower than about 250 per minute in association with second degree AV block, the pattern looks somewhat different from the classic "flutter" in that the baseline can be seen clearly between P waves, and the diagnosis of *"PAT with block"* must be considered, a diagnosis that differs from "flutter" only in atrial rate and has the clinical significance of suggesting digitalis toxicity perhaps 80% of the time.[80-82]

Sometimes the term *1:1 flutter*[77,475,607] is used to describe atrial tachycardia at a rate so rapid that one would expect there to be some degree of AV block, especially if AV block is seen intermittently. If more than one atrial focus is active, multifocal atrial tachycardia results[78,79,520] and is especially difficult to distinguish from atrial fibrillation.

The electrocardiographic diagnosis of *atrial fibrillation* (Figure 7-4) depends on recognition of evidence of fibrillation of the atria, i.e., an irregular baseline with fine undulations called "f" waves. When fibrillary waves are not readily apparent, their presence may be inferred from the observation that between no two pairs of QRS complexes in a given lead is the baseline the same. Irregularity of ventricular rhythm is not a criterion for the EKG diagnosis of atrial fibrillation, but it is typical and may be more difficult to recognize in the tracing than on physical examination. On physical examination one has not only the rhythm but also variations in volume of pulse, apical-radial pulse deficit, and the changing intensity of heart sounds to help him, but on the EKG he is dependent upon differences in cycle length. When the ventricular rate is very rapid or very slow this may call for especially careful measurement. It is possible to have atrial fibrillation with a perfectly regular ventricular rhythm as with

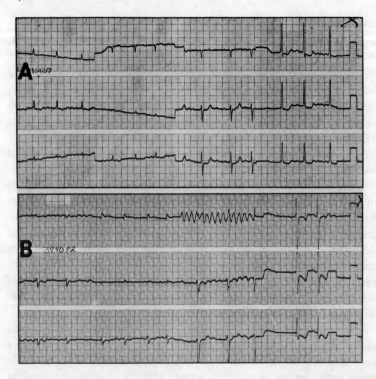

Figure 7-4. Atrial fibrillation. The EKG diagnosis is based on the configuration of the baseline between ventricular complexes, not just absence of P waves or irregularity of ventricular response. The amplitude of the grossly irregular deflections varies from large through small to almost unidentifiable. The lower tracing also shows left anterior hemiblock and ST-T abnormalities that probably mean left ventricular overload and/or anterior myocardial hypoxia. In the upper one the QRS is normal, and there are nonspecific ST-T abnormalities.

acceleration of a junctional pacemaker or when there is third degree AV block.

One may see in a single tracing places where atrial complexes can be identified at a rate of about 300 only to fade away into irregularity and then to be identifiable again later on. This can be called *impure flutter* or *flutter-fibrillation*,[16] but such detail has little if any clinical value. *Unilateral* atrial fibrillation has been reported.[84]

Atrial fibrillation is usually a consequence of mitral valve disease or coronary atherosclerosis, but it may be precipitated by other events that either stress the atrial wall, compromise its blood supply, or increase myocardial automaticity. Thyrotoxicosis may be an important factor and atrial fibrillation may appear following any thoracic procedure, with pericarditis, or it may even be familial.[596] It may be idiopathic and asymptomatic. It is rare in infants but may be a complication of an atrial septal defect. It is the only chronic cardiac arrhythmia compatible with health and may persist for many years. It may be seen without other evidence of heart disease or other electrocardiographic abnormality. The ventricular rate with atrial fibrillation covers the same range as that found with a sinus mechanism, between about 40 and 200 per minute. The two important clinical consequences of atrial fibrillation are thrombosis in the ineffectively contracting chambers, and the potential for embolism that this produces, and lessening of the pumping efficiency of the heart as a result of loss of presystolic injection of blood into the ventricles from the atria. If the heart is otherwise healthy, atrial fibrillation may be asymptomatic and require no treatment at all. Whether digitalis, quinidine, or another agent is called for depends upon the larger clinical setting.

Default Atrial Mechanisms

Electrocardiographic terminology provides no standard designation for slow mechanisms arising in the atria by default, but they do occur. They may originate in either atrium, are characterized by rates of the order of 50 to 70 per minute, and probably are covered by such terms as *left atrial* or *upper junctional* mechanisms; the language does not include "atrial bradycardia" but it would be logical.

AV Junctional Mechanisms

Mechanisms characterized by QRS complexes of supraventricular origin and retrograde P waves have been assumed traditionally to arise in the AV node and have been called "nodal rhythms." The usefulness of this term has not been modified much, but evidence that the AV node itself probably does not initiate impulses[85] has made it at least controversial, and it has been replaced for practical purposes by the designation "junctional" to include the area from low in the atria to the bifurcation of the bundle of His.[93,99,487]

Isolated "mainstem" premature contractions can originate in this area,[86,87] as may usurping and default mechanisms at rates between 40 and 200 per minute. All have normal (i.e., supraventricular) QRSs and retrograde P waves or no identifiable atrial activity. Retrograde depolarization of the atria is recognized by P waves that are negative in leads 2, 3, and F and usually negative in lead I and positive in aVR (Figure 7-5).

If the impulse arises low in an atrium, and this apparently occurs more commonly in the left atrium than in the right, the atria are depolarized before the ventricles and P precedes QRS — the PR interval is usually short,[57,73,88-95,455] *coronary sinus, left atrial, upper nodal,* or *upper junctional* mechanism. When the pacemaker lies near the center of the junctional area, P and QRS are assumed to be inscribed simultaneously, and the P is not identifiable, the classic *midnodal, or midjunctional*, mechanism. If the impulse arises low in the junctional area, presumably in the bundle of His itself,[96] the ventricles are depolarized before the atria and the retrograde P follows the QRS, a *low nodal or low junctional* mechanism. Contour and timing of the P and QRS in these mechanisms are influenced by varying degrees of antegrade and retrograde conduction delay and may not be explicable on the basis of anatomy alone.[97]

In summary, three types of electrocardiographic complexes are identifiable as arising in the AV junction. The QRS-T is normal in all of them. A beat originating in the center of the area, the classic nodal beat, shows no P wave at all. Beats originating high in the junction, probably actually in an atrium, are recognized by a retrograde P preceding the QRS, and a retrograde P follows the QRS in beats that originate low in the junction. Upper junctional mechanisms are fairly common and occur in the absence of evidence of heart disease, merging with sinus arrhythmia in their significance; lower ones are relatively rare and are more likely to be associated with disease. Slow (below about 50 per minute) junctional mechanisms are common with third-degree AV block; rapid (greater than about 50), or "accelerated," ones are seen with digitalis excess, febrile states, or inflammatory disease of the myocardium. When a junctional pacemaker functions at approximately sinus rate and AV conduction is normal, the PR varies — "isorhythmic dissociation."[560,655]

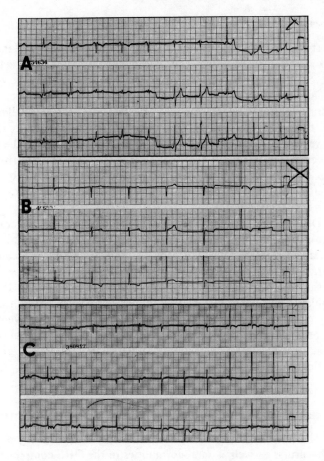

Figure 7-5. Junctional (or nodal) mechanisms. In the top tracing P is negative in leads 2, 3, F, and V_1 and V_6, i.e., the atria are depolarized from a point below and to the left of normal, presumably low in an atrium or high in a vaguely defined "junctional" area. They have a symmetric, V-shaped contour and are associated with a short PR interval. In the middle tracing no atrial activity is identifiable, and it is assumed that the atria and ventricles are depolarized simultaneously and P waves do not show. Other explanations are possible, but this is called a midjunctional mechanism. In the lower tracing the retrograde P follows the QRS in the first four beats and is interpreted as having arisen from a point closer to the ventricles than to the atria, a low junctional focus, probably in the His bundle. P precedes QRS in the last three beats and is probably of sinus origin; it is not identifiable with confidence in the others.

Supraventricular Tachycardia of Uncertain Origin

It is not unusual to find a tracing with normal ventricular complexes at a very rapid rate but without identifiable atrial activity. There will be a question as to whether a P is written while the ventricles are being repolarized, so that the single deflection between QRS complexes should be interpreted as a "PT," and often one will not be able to decide (Figure 7-1). The important thing to recognize is that the ventricular complexes are of supraventricular origin. If the pacemaker cannot be identified, the tracing is said to show *supraventricular tachycardia of uncertain origin,* and an opinion as to which specific diagnosis is most likely may be added. Atrial tachycardia may occur without P waves.[519]

Distortion of the QRS complex in some beats, often several in a series, is common in all supraventricular tachycardias, usually in a pattern of right bundle branch block. This is a result of inconstant characteristics of refractoriness and is called *ventricular aberration,* a transient abnormality of intraventricular conduction. It may simulate ventricular tachycardia, either paroxysmal or consistent, very closely. Differentiation between ventricular and supraventricular origin of these beats is of obvious prognostic importance but often depends upon information other than that in the electrocardiogram.

Special Characteristics of the AV Junction Related to Arrhythmias

The junctional area is of complex importance in the genesis of tachycardias as well as in abnormalities of the QRS complex,[97] and recordings from the His bundle and other parts of the intracardiac conduction system have helped to elucidate some of its characteristics.[100-102] The terminology is complex and less than standard[557] and often fails to make clear the difference between description and interpretation.

The concept of *concealed conduction,*[103,104,425,426,461] incomplete penetration of atrial impulses into the AV node, has been offered as a part of the explanation for the varying rate and rhythm of ventricular response to atrial fibrillation and for prolongation of the PR in postextrasystolic beats.[105] *Entrance block,*[429] analogous to other forms of AV block, is said to exist when impulses from above do not penetrate the AV node at all, necessitating a pacemaker in the junction to drive the ventricles, and may be seen as a result of digitalis toxicity.[106] *Exit block* is a fairly complex concept implying failure of an impulse to be transmitted from its site of origin to surrounding tissues.[107,108,417,460]

The old view that electrical impulses traverse the AV pathways in one direction only, from above downward, has changed. While it is true that most of the time propagation is antegrade only, this apparently is related to refractory period rather than any intrinsic "one-way" characteristic of the tissue itself. *Longitudinal dissociation*[97,109-111,412,546] and *dual conduction*[111,112] with the normal AV pathways, perhaps together with any of the various paranodal pathways (see page 84), may explain *reentry*,[33,71,72,109,412,435,535] *echo*, or *reciprocal* beating. An impulse may be transmitted from the ventricles retrograde to depolarize the atria and then, if refractory periods permit, reenter the ventricles, and so on in a repetitive fashion, a possible explanation for either paroxysmal or sustained episodes of tachycardia. The beat that initiates this response may be of either atrial or ventricular origin.[98,109,110,111,113-118]

The idea of a *supernormal* period of AV conduction is logical but controversial. It implies that just as there are absolute and relative refractory phases of reactivity of nerve and muscle following depolarization, there is also a brief phase of hyperresponsiveness. This hypothesis is invoked sometimes to explain unexpected conductivity in the intracardiac conduction system and sometimes in problems of irritability.[119-122,425,427]

VENTRICULAR MECHANISMS

As in the atria, abnormalities of impulse formation in the ventricles may be either usurping or default (Figure 7-6).

Premature Ventricular Contractions

Isolated beats arising from a ventricular pacemaker are called *premature ventricular contractions* (PVC) and are identified by prematurity, a broad (0.12 sec or more), bizarre QRS, and the absence of a related P wave[428] (Figure 7-8). The configuration is a function of the location of the ectopic focus, those originating in the left ventricle having the form generally of right bundle branch block and those originating in the right ventricle that of left bundle branch

SINUS WITH PVC's

VENTRICULAR
TACHYCARDIA

VENTRICULAR
FIBRILLATION

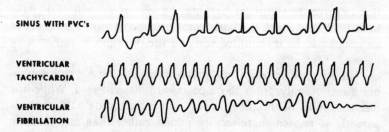

Figure 7-6. Ventricular mechanisms. PVCs = premature ventricular contractions.

block.[123] The ST-T complex associated with PVCs is modified proportionately, and the premature beat typically is followed by a compensatory pause, i.e., the first postextrasystolic beat occurs at the same time that it would have had there not been a PVC — without interruption of the basic sinus rhythm. Occasional PVCs apparently occur in everyone and when asymptomatic may be considered within normal limits; when they are frequent, though, a designation that calls for judgment and depends to some extent upon the symptoms they produce and the clinical setting in which they occur, arise from multiple foci, are of left ventricular origin, or when the myocardium is not normal, they are more likely to be of serious import.[124] Their appearance in a bigeminal pattern, coupled, occurring with a fixed relation to conducted beats, is of little clinical significance. There is a tradition that PVCs coinciding with the "vulnerable period" of ventricular repolarization (near the peak or on the downstroke of the T wave) are likely to initiate ventricular automaticity, but there is reason to doubt this.[544,569] Three or more consecutive PVCs define ventricular tachycardia. *Interpolated* PVCs are sandwiched between two normal beats without breaking the regular rhythm. They are true "extrasystoles" but have no specific significance. The PR interval of the first postextrasystolic beat may be prolonged, and this may be explained by such concepts as concealed retrograde conduction. *End-diastolic* PVCs occur after a normal P wave but before the impulse has had time to reach the ventricles; the presence of a P at the expected time may make the prematurity of the beat less noticeable. The PR interval is very short, though, and there is no causal relationship between the P and the

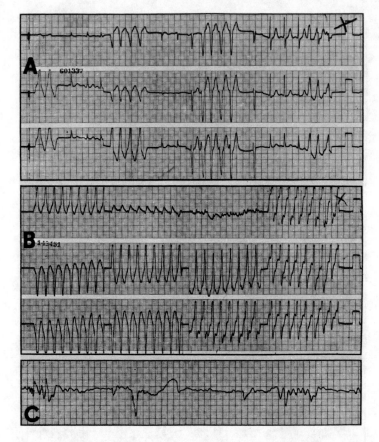

Figure 7-7. Ventricular tachycardia and fibrillation. In the top tracing the basic mechanism is sinus at a rate of 120, and there are brief paroxysms of ventricular activity at a rate of about 200, irregular rhythm, and inconstant QRS contour; in the middle tracing the QRS rate is a little above 200, and the rhythm is regular and the contour consistent. In both of these the pacemaker is probably in a ventricle, but alternative explanations invoking combinations of supraventricular pacemakers and intraventricular conduction defects are possible. Diagnosis of ventricular tachycardia at a level of confidence sufficient to justify therapeutic action almost always requires more information than that provided in the tracing alone. The bottom strip shows the wavy, inconstant pattern of ventricular fibrillation. Ventricular tachycardia and fibrillation form a continuum and distinction between them is often arbitrary and of little import. Ventricular bradycardia, a default mechanism traditionally called "idioventricular rhythm" also exists.

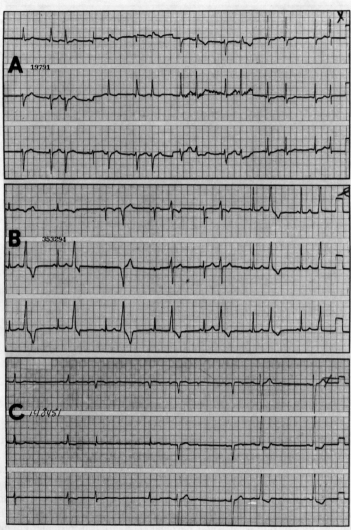

Figure 7-8. Bigeminy. Bigeminy designates pairing of beats. It may be due to increased automaticity of an ectopic pacemaker, second-degree AV block, or other mechanisms. In the top tracing it is caused by premature atrial contractions (atrial bigeminy); the middle one, PVC (ventricular bigeminy); and in the bottom one to second-degree AV block. Another basis for bigeminy is slowing of the sinus node with escape by a slower pacemaker in the junctional area followed by a beat of sinus origin, and so on — "escape-capture" bigeminy.

QRS except to the degree that there is some fusion (see Fusion Beats, page 95).

If the ventricular focus fires repetitively at a rapid rate, usually between 160 and 200, the mechanism is called *ventricular tachycardia* (Figure 7-7). This is almost always a complication of serious myocardial disease, often acute myocardial infarction, and is a major medical emergency. Ideally it can be recognized by the rapid rate, slightly varying rhythm, and broad, bizarre QRS complexes. Differentiation from supraventricular tachycardia with bundle branch block or ventricular aberration is important because of the prognostic implications, but sometimes is not possible on the basis of the electrocardiogram alone, especially if there is no control tracing. The QRS rhythm with ventricular tachycardia is more likely to vary perceptibly than with a supraventricular one, and ideally one should be able to demonstrate P wave occurring independently at a slower rate, as well as occasional fusion beats, in the former.[125,464] Very rarely paroxysmal ventricular tachycardia occurs in the absence of other evidence of heart disease.[126]

Occasionally one sees QRS complexes of ventricular origin at a rate greater than the usual escape rate of 30 or 40 but less than the 160 or more expected with typical ventricular tachycardia, nearer the dominant or sinus rate. The terminology by which this should be designated is not standard and includes such expressions as *slow ventricular tachycardia, recurrent paroxysmal ventricular tachycardia, accelerated idioventricular rhythm,* and *ventricular tachysystole.*[104,130-132] Its clinical significance is less ominous than that of ventricular tachycardia in the ordinary sense.

Bidirectional tachycardia is a rare finding characterized by broad, bizarre QRS complexes of two configurations alternating with each other.[432] One explanation is that this is due to alternating block of anterior and posterior divisions of the left bundle in the presence of right bundle branch block.[127]

Ventricular fibrillation is a common mechanism of death. It used to be an electrocardiographic rarity about which nothing could be done and recorded only when a tracing happened to be in progress at the time of death. Its recognition is easy, though, with modern monitoring facilities and is of obvious importance because there are means of reverting it and practical methods of cardiopulmonary resuscitation. It produces a chaotic tracing with no individuallly identifiable complexes (see Figure 7-7) but merges with ventricular tachycardia. It may be a paroxysmal phenomenon lasting only a few seconds and reverting spontaneously, but usually is a clear indication for electrical intervention. It has been reported to occur intermittently in otherwise normal young people[128] and may be the basis for syncope in patients with a *long QT-U syndrome* (see page 167).

When a pacemaker in the ventricles drives them regularly at about 30 per minute, an *idioventricular mechanism* is present.

There is such a thing, of course, as literal *cardiac standstill*. It is manifest by a perfectly flat trace with no evidence of electrical activity. It is encountered rarely and is an indication for the use of artifical pacing if this can be begun within seconds after its onset. Sometimes a simple blow to the chest with the fist will elicit an electrical impulse and produce a beat.[129]

Artificial Pacemakers

The patterns produced by artificial ventricular pacemakers vary with the position of the pacing electrode.[370,371] and the characteristics of the specific make and model. The two things seen in the tracing are the pacemaker stimulus itself and the QRS it produces. The pacemaker stimulus appears as an instantaneous spike that may be positive or negative, great or small, and may be found in any lead depending upon the location of the electrode(s) within the heart. The QRS contour is determined by the position of the electrode also, having the characteristics of right bundle branch block when the stimulus is applied to the left ventricle and of left bundle branch block when applied to the right. Artificial pacemakers can produce very complicated arrhythmias by interaction with intrinsic pacemakers.[404] Distinction should be made between firing and capturing: a pacemaker may fire regularly or irregularly and capture appropriately or not at all. Details of analysis require knowledge of the type of pacemaker. Sometimes the trace may be so distorted by a large pacemaker stimulus that it looks like a QRS; the artifact, though, will not be followed by a T as would a QRS complex.

Miscellaneous

Bigeminy (literally, two twins) refers to pairing of beats, the occurrence of beats relatively close to each other and separated from the next two by a pause. It may be due to premature contractions (supraventricular or ventricular) after each sinus beat,[7,8] second degree AV block with 3:2 conduction, or other combinations. Escape-capture bigeminy is an unusual form in which a period of sinus inactivity results in escape of a lower pacemaker after which a normally conducted sinus beat occurs promptly, another pause follows, escape again, and so on in such a sequence that the conducted beat is the second of the pair. To say only that a patient has bigeminy is not enough; the mechanism by which the beats are paired must be stated. It makes a difference in prognosis and management whether the bigeminy is due to premature discharge of an ectopic focus implying irritability, to AV block implying depression of function, or to compensatory mechanisms.

The concept of *parasystole*[75,133-135,431,656] is that there is an ectopic pacemaker initiating beats at a rate different from that of the sinus node and somehow protected from depolarization by the sinus beats. Ventricular tachycardia as described above can be defined as an example of this, but the term usually implies complexes initiated by the ectopic focus at a rate slower than the dominant one. Ventricular parasystole is the form most frequently recognized but it occurs in the atria, too.[75] It produces a pattern that may be hard to differentiate from ordinary PVCs unless suspected. It probably is not rare if looked for in tracings that are long enough to permit its identification, and may have no more clinical significance than ordinary premature ventricular contractions.[418]

Supernormality of ventricular excitability may explain some ectopic beats in response to what otherwise would be an inadequate stimulus.[667]

CHAPTER VIII

Abnormalities of AV Conduction

In the normal heart the only way that electrical impulses originating in the sinus node or atria can reach the ventricles is through the AV node and the His bundle and its branches. The rate of conduction of this system ranges from very slow in the node itself to very fast in the specialized His-Purkinje tissue with the overall result that the duration of the PR interval in normals is not more than about 0.20 second. When impulses are generated in the sinus node or atria more rapidly than the rate at which the junctional system is capable of transmitting them, AV block is present.* This disproportion may exist in varying degree, ranging from simple prolongation of AV conduction time through failure to conduct some beats to complete interruption of electrical continuity between atria and ventricles — first- second- and third-degree, or complete, AV block (Figure 8-1). It may reflect abnormally rapid atrial activity and/or impairment of conductivity in the AV node, His bundle, or bundle branches; it may be retrograde or antegrade. Some special features of AV junctional tissues indicated in the preceeding chapter are relevant to the discussion that follows.

First-Degree AV Block

The length of the PR interval is a measure of the time required for excitation to traverse the AV junction. It varies inversely with the heart rate. First-degree AV block is present when there is delay in

---

*AV block is sometimes called "heart block," a term that is imprecise because it logically applies equally well to intraventricular block.

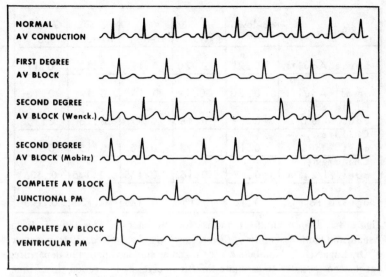

Figure 8-1. Atrioventricular (AV) block. Wenck. = Wenckebach.
PM = pacemaker.

transmission through the junctional tissue and is recognized by prolongation of the PR interval. Normal values are tabulated in Figure
8-2; the upper limit is about 0.20 sec in an adult with ventricular rate
less than 100 per minute. Neither P nor QRS-T is changed in first
degree AV block, and there is still one P wave for each QRS. It
should be emphasized that the PR should not be estimated any closer
than 0.02 sec by inspection, and that the first-degre AV block does
not necessarily mean disease.[433]

Second-Degree AV Block

If delay in conduction is such that not all impulses that reach the
AV node from above get through to the ventricles, but some do and
all ventricular complexes are derived from them, second-degree AV
block* is present. The electrocardiogram shows fewer ventricular

---

*Second-degree block was recognized in 1899 by Wenckebach[139] whose ob-
servations were based on mechanical recordings of jugular and arterial
pulses. His findings were confirmed with similar techniques by Hay[140] in
1906 and electrocardiographically by Mobitz in 1924.[141]

RATE	Below 70	71–90	91–110	111–130	Above 130
Large Adults	0.21	0.20	0.19	0.18	0.17
Small Adults	0.20	0.19	0.18	0.17	0.16
Children, ages 14 to 17	0.19	0.18	0.17	0.16	0.15
Children, ages 7 to 13	0.18	0.17	0.16	0.15	0.14
Children, ages 1 1/2 to 6	0.17	0.165	0.155	0.145	0.135
Children, ages 0 to 1 1/2	0.16	0.15	0.145	0.135	0.125

Figure 8-2. Upper limits of normal for PR interval. This table is from Asham and Hull, *Essentials of Electrocardiography*, 2nd. ed., 1941, courtesy of Dr. Edgar Hull. Numbers can be taken as standard points of departure, but it is not possible to estimate the PR interval by inspection closer than about 0.02 sec.

complexes than atrial and the ventricular complexes are all of supraventricular origin.

There are two types of second-degree AV block. In the common form, *Wenckebach* (Type I), the PR interval increases progressively until a QRS complex is dropped and the cycle is repeated — Wenckebach periods.[142] In the other form, *Mobitz* (Type II), a QRS complex is dropped without warning, either regularly or irregularly.[143] Both types were described by all the pioneers in the field, but Type I is traditionally known by Wenckebach's name and Type II as Mobitz II. Wenckebach block is common as a result of digitalis, atherosclerosis, inflammatory disease, or recent inferior myocardial infarction. It is often transient and generally has a good prognosis. The Mobitz II form is relativey uncommon, more likely than the Wenckebach to be followed by complete block, and usually has an ominous significance.[434]

Third-Degree AV Block

When AV block is complete, none of the impulses from above gets through the junctional tissue, and the ventricles must be driven by a lower focus. The electrocardiogram shows atrial activity (be it of sinus origin, atrial tachycardia, or atrial fibrillation) bearing no predictable relation to the QRS complexes that are occurring at a regular rhythm and a rate slower than the atria.

When the pacemaker driving the ventricles is above the bifurcation of the bundle of His (junctional), QRS complexes are narrow, of normal configuration (unless there is also an intraventricular conduction defect), and occur at rate of about 40–50. This is likely to be stable while it lasts and to resolve spontaneously. It is seen commonly when Av block complicates inferior infarction. When the pacemaker for the ventricles is within the ventricles themselves (idioventricular), QRS complexes are broad, slurred, of bizarre configuration, and occur at a rate of about 30 per minute. This is likely to be an unstable mechanism with a poor prognosis.[145,146]

A complete electrocardiographic diagnosis must name the pacemaker for the atria, indicate the presence of complete AV block, and identify the pacemaker driving the ventricles, e.g., sinus mechanism with complete AV block and an idioventricular pacemaker.

Discussion

The electrocardiographic diagnosis of AV block is not difficult if the tracing is long enough for adequate study. Organization of the information in the form of a diagram (Figure 8-3) is helpful. It makes no difference which lead is used as long as both Ps and QRSs are identifiable. Lead 2 is usually satisfactory, but sometimes V₁ or V₂ is better, and esophageal leads or intra-atrial leads may be used if the P cannot be identified otherwise. A good technician will recognize a disorder of AV conduction while the tracing is being recorded and make a long strip of an appropriate lead. the degree of block diagnosed should describe the tracing as a whole and not an isolated group of complexes.

AV block may result from a combination of lesions in the IV conduction system or from a single lesion in the His bundle or above, and recordings made directly from the His bundle and its branches have contributed to an understanding of this problem.[101]

Most AV block is the result of inflammatory disease, drugs (quinidine or digitalis), or anatomic lesions that are either idiopathic or result from coronary atherosclerosis.[138,148] Congenital block occurs, usually in association with other lesions such as an endocardial

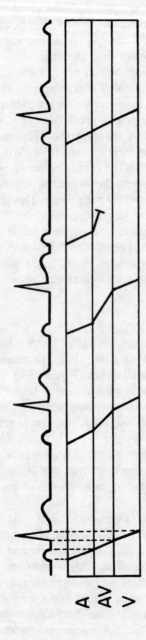

Figure 8-3. The AV diagram, or laddergram, a device for analysis of mechanism. The time of beginning of the P wave is noted on the top line and its end on the second one. Beginning of QRS is indicated on the third line and its end on the bottom one. When the atrial and ventricular levels are connected, the slopes of the connecting lines indicate the duration of AV connection. This method of analysis of mechanism is older than electrocardiography itself.[698] It helps to emphasize that the relation between P and QRS is always and necessarily a matter of judgment. More complex diagrams can be set up for SA conduction, subdivisions of AV conduction, and other variations that are possible.

cushion defect or corrected transposition of the great vessels, but this is uncommon.[147,407,408] The fixed, chronic, complete AV block of elderly patients with or without Stokes-Adams attacks usually is idiopathic. Each of these mechanisms may produce any degree of block, but complete block as a result of drugs is rare. The electrocardiogram shows only the block and does not indicate its etiology.[148]

Accelerated Junctional Pacemaker ("interference dissociation")

The word "dissociation" is not a very specialized one and has no specific significance in electrocardiography. To speak of AV dissociation is to imply that beating of the atria and ventricles is imperfectly correlated, or associated. When dissociation is complete, there must be two pacemakers, one for the atria and one for the ventricles. *Complete AV block* with one pacemaker above the block and another below it is an example of AV dissociation in this broad sense of the word; another, the one usually implied, is the presence in the AV junction of a pacemaker initiating impulses at a rate faster than that of the sinus node. When this occurs, the ventricles will almost always be refractory at the time of arrival of the impulse from the sinus node, but sometimes they will be responsive and a normally conducted beat will appear. This beat will be premature and produce a refractory state that blocks the next beat from above. This type of dissociation is a subject of some confusion in the literature, not because of any inherent difficulty in understanding it but because of the use of different names for it, the most logical one being acceleration of a junctional pacemaker with *interference dissociation*.[153-155]

Interference dissociation is a relatively unusual finding and of itself not very disturbing. Its common causes are rheumatic fever and other inflammatory diseases, coronary artery disease, and digitalis effect, and its significance is that of the underlying processes. When both sinus and junctional pacemakers are active at about the same rate, the relation between P and QRS varies. There may be a very short PR interval or P and QRS may merge in a stepwise fashion. This is called *isorhythmic dissociation*.[560,655] Its clinical significance is a function largely of the rate; if slow, it is simply a normal response of a junctional pacemaker when the sinus pacemaker falls below its inherent rate; if rapid, it may indicate acceleration of a junctional pacemaker.

VENTRICULAR PREEXCITATION

If the electrical signal from the atria bypasses the AV node, entering the ventricular myocardium by way of one or a combination of several possible paranodal pathways, i.e., preexcitation,[439] AV conduction time will be shortened, and the contour of the initial part of the QRS complex may be changed. The classic example of this, described in 1930 by Wolff, Parkinson, and White[179] and known by their names, is based on the anomalous presence of specialized conduction tissue, a bundle of Kent, connecting atria with ventricles at a peripheral site.[180,184,1895] The pattern produced by Wolff-Parkinson-White (WPW) syndrome represents a fusion beat (see page 95) and is characterized by an initial slur that results from abnormally early onset of depolarization at some point in the myocardium other than the junctional area, preexcitation. When the mechanism is sinus the PR is shortened to the same extent that the QRS is widened by this "delta wave" (Figure 8-4);[696] the time from the beginning of P to the end of the QRS remains normal. The QRS pattern may be divided into two groups on the basis of the orientation of the early part of the complex; in group A this is directly anteriorly and either superiorly or inferiorly, and in group B to the left, posteriorly, and either superiorly or inferiorly,[21] but there is no clinical value differentiating between the two types except in the rare cases in which surgical intervention is anticipated.[406]

The Wolff-Parkinson-White syndrome is uncommon, with its incidence estimated at about 0.15%,[185] and may be found in any age group but is seen most frequently in young adults. It has no prognostic significance other than the fact that it is associated with a high incidence of paroxysmal supraventricular tachycardia.[180,186] Its greatest importance lies in the fact that it may be misinterpreted as evidence of heart disease. It may stimulate bundle branch block with which it may coexist[187] or, if the rate is fast, ventricular tachycardia,[188] and it may either simulate or obscure EKG evidence of myocardial infarction.[189-192] It may be persistent or remarkably labile, present in some tracings and not in others or even in alternate beats in the same tracing. In some cases it may be made to appear or disappear in response to changes in vagus tone, exercise, position, or even deep breathing.[180]

In rare instances of persistence of debilitating tachycardia in pa-

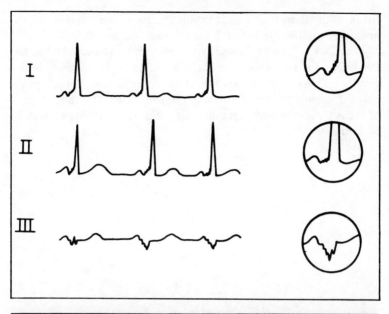

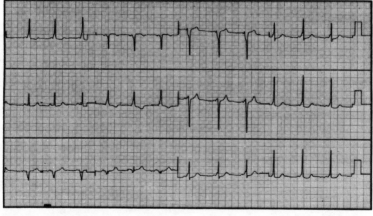

Figure 8-4. Ventricular preexcitation. The Wolff-Parkinson-White syndrome. The important abnormality is deformity of the initial part of the QRS as a result of abnormally early beginning of ventricular depolarization via an anomalous electrical communication between atria and ventricles; shortening of PR is incidental.

tients with abnormal preexcitation, surgical interruption of the anomalous pathways has stopped the tachycardia.[193,194,406]

The *Lown-Ganong-Levine syndrome* can be suspected when the PR interval is very short and the QRS is normal, especially in patients with paroxysms of rapid heart action by history, but it is probably impossible to identify from the tracing alone. It implies bypass of the AV node by way of anomalous pathways other than a Bundle of Kent.[181,648-650]

CHAPTER IX

Disorders of Intraventricular Conduction

Impairment of intraventricular conduction produces changes in QRS orientation, duration, and/or contour; specific patterns depend upon the location and extent of the lesion.

Right Bundle Branch Block

If propagation of electrical impulses is impeded in the right bundle branch while remaining normal in the left, excitation of myocardium supplied by the right bundle is delayed and that on the left is not. This produces changes in QRS duration (prolongation to 0.12 sec or more) and contour (Figure 9-1), but does not necessarily affect orientation, axis.

Consider two leads, one on the right side of the precordium and one on the left, V_1 and V_6. In the normal heart, forces generated during depolarization of the interventricular septum initiate the QRS complex and are directed anteriorly and to the right, giving rise to a small deflection that is an R in V_1 and a Q in V_6. The impulse then proceeds outward from the subendocardium simultaneously over the remainder of both ventricles and produces forces which, as a whole, are directed to the left, down, and posteriorly, giving rise to an S in V_1 and an R in V_6. When the right bundle branch is blocked, depolarization of the septum is not changed substantially, and excitation of the left ventricle proceeds normally and ends in about 0.06-0.08 sec. During this time, the delayed wave front reaches the right ventricle by way of pathways other than normal and begins to produce forces directed anteriorly and to the right. The first part of the QRS complex is normal, but these late events, completed after depolarization of the left ventricle has finished, are reflected in a broad, abnormally shaped terminal deflection that is positive in

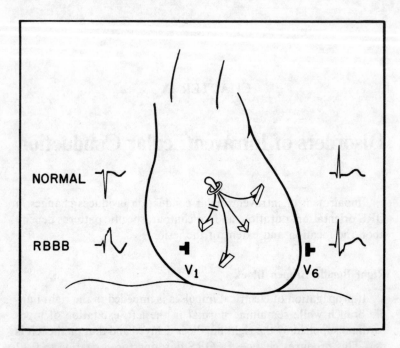

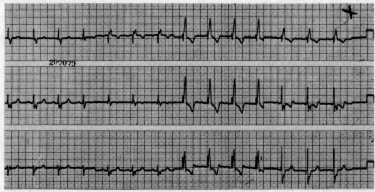

Figure 9-1. Right bundle branch block. Depolarization of the right (anterior) ventricle occurs late and over an abnormal route, producing typical deformity of the terminal portion of the QRS by forces directed anteriorly and somewhat to the right.

leads from the right and negative in those from the left. The delay, or block, may be slight or considerable and details of QRS configuration vary, but terminal abnormality directed to the right and anteriorly is the hallmark and is seen best in a right precordial lead where there is small initial upstroke followed by downstroke and, finally, a broad, slurred, positive wave. Left precordial leads in right bundle branch block end with a broad, slurred negative deflection. When the picture is less than typical, the pattern of right bundle branch block merges with that of right ventricular enlargement (especially right ventricular enlargement due to diastolic overload as with an atrial septal defect) on the one hand and with normal on the other. An rSr V_1 may fall into either of these categories; it is not by itself an abnormal finding[555] and to call it "incomplete" right bundle branch block adds little.

Left Bundle Branch Block

Unlike the right bundle branch that can be thought of as a single strand through most it its course (a wire) the left one begins to branch very shortly below the bifurcation of the His bundle and is more like a cable with frayed and widely spread ends. The pattern of right bundle branch block varies in detail but always includes a broad, slurred, terminal component directed anteriorly and usually to the right; left bundle branch block is less easily categorized (Figure 9-2). When the lesion is proximal enough, excitation of the interventricular septum proceeds from its right (anterior) aspect leftward and posteriorly. The QRS is prolonged to at least 0.12 sec, and is completely positive with more or less prominent notching and slurring throughout in leads whose positive pole is left, down, or back (1, aVL, V_6, and sometimes 2 and aVF). If the block is a little more distal, the initial part of the complex will be left intact.

"Incomplete" left bundle block[156-158] can be defined, but there is no generally accepted standard for it and the term has little value; identification of block of subdivisions of the system is more useful. Distal lesions produce more or less typical patterns of lesser degrees of deformity; left anterior hemiblock, left posterior hemiblock, and/ or block of an anterior septal fascicle. The principal abnormality produced by these fascicular blocks is one of orientation of the terminal part of the QRS (axis deviation). Duration and/or contour

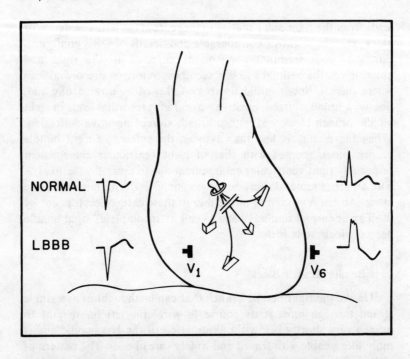

NORMAL

LBBB

V_1

V_6

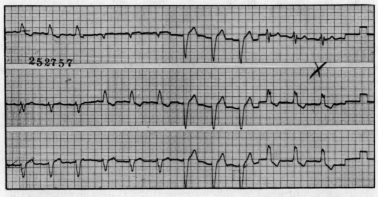

252757

Figure 9-2. Left bundle branch block. Left bundle branch block represents a continuum; when proximal enough, a characteristic picture is produced with deformity of the whole QRS complex directed to the left and back.

may or may not be abnormal; they form a continuum between normal and "complete" left bundle branch block,[508] and left bundle branch block is not always associated with left axis deviation.[660]

Block of Subdivisions of the Left Bundle Branch

One of the most important developments in electrocardiography in the past few years has been a better understanding of the intraventricular conduction system and the electrocardiographic manifestations of impairment of its function. The early work of Drs. Grant,[159] Pryor and Blount,[160] and Watt, et al[161] should be noted; Dr. James' studies of the intraventricular conduction system are of fundamental importance;[507] and the contributions of Dr. Rosenbaum have been especially influential.[151,164,451] Impairment of conduction in the anterosuperior division of the bundle branch, the posteroinferior one, and, perhaps, an intermediate or septal one can be recognized.[534,540,543] The existence of these fascicles as discrete anatomic entities is putative at best, but in the present state of knowledge they are reasonable and useful hypotheses to explain electrocardiographic findings that are enigmatic otherwise. The nomenclature is controversial but not very important; fascicular block is more logical, since it would not limit the system to two components, but hemiblock is the name more widely used. By whatever name, the implication is local conduction delay, a lesion in the ventricular wall.

Left Anterior Hemiblock

Ever since the very early days of electrocardiography it has been recognized that the mean QRS in the frontal plane, the axis, is farther counter clockwise in some people than in others and that this statistical abnormality, "left axis deviation" (see page 159), may or may not be associated with clinical evidence of heart disease. This *finding* has been treated sometimes as if it were a diagnosis, an example of failure to differentiate between description and interpretation, and an enigma that seems to have been a major basis for Dr. Rosenbaum's studies.[164] Let us consider possible explanations for it.

If all the electrical forces generated during depolarization of the ventricles are lumped together, expressed as a net value, and represented as a line beginning at the center of Einthoven's reference frame, the direction of this vector, or "axis," can be measured easily, expressed in degrees, and the range of normal established. Many studies have shown that in subjects without heart disease this lies between about −30° and +105° with a limit of tolerance of about 15° at each end. Values counterclockwise to this, abnormal by definition, may be the result of one or more of four things: increase in forces directed leftward and upward, loss of forces directed downward and rightward, change in the route over which the ventricular myocardium is depolarized, or change in the electrical properties of the system invalidating Einthoven's premises.

Increase in forces to the left and cephalad would result from disproportionate left ventricular hypertrophy. This is logical and must occur, but left axis deviation does not correlate significantly with left ventricular overload and is not an important feature in its diagnosis[294] (see pages 91 and 127). Loss of forces directed caudad and to the right occurs with inferior myocardial scarring and does indeed often produce left axis deviation, but it also produces change in QRS contour and abnormalities of contour always takes precedence over those of mean; when an infarct is diagnosed little attention is paid to the axis as such. There is one common clinical setting in which Einthoven's premises are not operative and which influences the direction of the QRS — pulmonary emphysema. Pulmonary emphysema replaces tissue with air, and the electrical properties of air are not the same as those of the other components of the volume conductor (the torso); left axis deviation is not rare in patients with pulmonary emphysema without heart disease.

There is a group of patients whose QRS is directed to between −45° and −90°, though, and in whom none of these explanations is applicable. It can be hypothesized that in this group changes have occurred in the His-Purkinje system so that activation of the anterior ventricular myocardium takes place over a route different from normal. That such an explanation is reasonable, even probable, is supported by demonstration of subdivisios of the left bundle branch.[164,507] Anatomic study of such small structures is exceedingly difficult and there are differences of opinion as to details of the findings, the extent to which the fascicles are functionally distinct, and the terminology that should be used to describe them. That there are such subdivisions, though, and that their function is as postulated is supported by several observations. Scarification of the ventricular myocardium of primates in areas predicated to include antero-superior ramifications of the left bundle branch has been shown to produce the expected electrocardiographic changes,[161] counter-clockwise displacement of the frontal QRS has been described dur-ing left anterior descending coronary artery opacification,[167] and transient "left axis deviation" has been documented during graded exercise testing[531] as well as in association with chest pain typical of angina.

What all this amounts to is that marked counterclockwise direc-tion of the frontal QRS in the absence of some other explanation for it can be interpreted as evidence of impairment of conduction in the anterosuperior ramification of the left bundle branch, i.e., left anterior hemiblock or left anterior fascicular block. The electro-cardiographic criteria for its diagnosis are a QRS complex with nor-mal initial contour (usually a small Q in lead 1 and a small R in 2 and 3) and a mean direction (axis) at least as far counterclockwise as about −60° (and not past −90°). QRS duration may be prolonged, but this is not necessary for the diagnosis (Figure 9-3).

The clinical significance of left anterior hemiblock depends upon its cause. IV conduction defects in general imply structural change. They may result from any process that produces myocardial scar-ring. Atherosclerosis is high on this list, of course, but other possi-bilities include congenital anomaly, trauma, infection, infiltrative disease, edema, drug effect or metabolic change, and idiopath-ic[661-663]; proof of the cause is rarely forthcoming. When present as an isolated finding, left anterior hemiblock probably means that there is patchy fibrosis or idiopathic abnormality in the myocardium[451] and has little significance in itself. The concomitant diagnosis of anter-ior myocardial infarction and left anterior hemiblock is easy and logical, but it must be kept in mind that left anterior hemiblock may simulate an anterior infarct[511,538,691] or obscure one.[164,628] Inferior infarction and left anterior hemiblock may coexist, but to diagnose both from a single tracing involves internal conflict. Recognition of one depends upon abnormality of the initial forces while the defini-tion of the other requires that they be normal. Left axis deviation seen with left ventricular hypertrophy may or may not be due to left anterior hemiblock related to patchy fibrosis rather than to an in-crease in forces originating in the hypertrophied ventricle, and

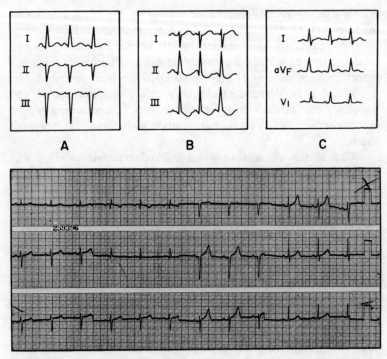

Figure 9-3. Left anterior hemiblock, left posterior hemiblock, and anterior conduction delay. The tracing shows a classic example of left anterior hemiblock, and there may be an old anterior myocardial infarct, too. Left posterior hemiblock, though it must exist, overlaps normal so widely that it is seldom diagnosed; the concept of isolated delay of conduction anteriorly in the left ventricle is less widely recognized than the other two but probably has equal validity.

pulmonary emphysema may simulate left anterior hemiblock by invalidating Einthoven's premises. Potassium toxicity may produce a picture inseparable from left anterior hemiblock.[443,516]

Left Posterior Hemiblock

Left posterior hemiblock must exist but is seen less frequently than anterior, presumably becuase of the dual blood supply to the posteroinferior region of the septum from both left and right coronary arteries and the diffuse nature of the left posterior subdivision.[164,169] Criteria for its diagnosis are a mean frontal QRS more clockwise than +105° and, usually, a small initial R1 and Q2 and Q3. As with anterior hemiblock it may result from anything that impairs conduction, but distinction from normal on the one hand and from right ventricular enlargement on the other is so arbitrary that the diagnosis is rarely proposed except as an explanation for some of the findings in a subset of right bundle branch block.

Anterior Conduction Delay

There is reason to suspect that an anterior septal subdivision of the left bundle branch exists as a functional entity and must be included along with dorsal infarction, right ventricular hypertrophy, and right bundle branch block in the differential diagnosis of abnormal anterior direction of QRS.[534,540,541,543,580,623] If there is such a fascicle, the "hemiblock" and "trifascicular" terminology is not accurate, but there are many examples in electrocardiography of nomenclature that on retrospective analysis is not logical.

Combinations of Intraventricular Blocks, "Bifascicular Block"

Recognizing that right bundle branch block need not by itself produce "axis deviation,"[172] it is logical to suspect that marked left or right axis deviation of a QRS that shows the typical deformity of right bundle branch block would be the result of coexisting left anterior or posterior hemiblock, bifascicular block,[150,151] and the prognostic implication of bifascicular block in a trifascicular system is clear. This concept was emerging at the same time that means for control of the electrical activity of the heart were being developed, and the diagnosis of right bundle branch block in combination with left anterior or posterior hemiblock came to be considered by some an indication for implantation of a cardiac pacemaker even in the absence of symptoms. To prove that this is not appropriate would border on the impossible, but the consequences to the patient of such reasoning are so important that the hypothesis must be evaluated as carefully as possible. It presents two problems: first, is it logical, or possible, to make the diagnosis of block at two sites from a single set of data when the block in each instance distorts the terminal QRS forces selectively, and second even if it is accepted that this can be done, does the prognosis of asymptomatic patients with right bundle branch block and "left axis deviation" justify such major intervention?

Granted that the diagnosis of either right bundle branch block or left anterior hemiblock by itself is logical and meaningful, the anatomic premises underlying either would be invalidated for use in the diagnosis of the other by the presence of the first—i.e., right bundle branch block is recognized by abnormality of the terminal part of the QRS, and the diagnosis of left anterior hemiblock depends upon changes in the same portion of the complex. To say that one is present is to imply that the rules by which the other must be diagnosed are not operative. The diagnosis of bifascicular block from a single tracing represents a decision expressed in convincing words but depends upon estimation of very, very small values that are tenuous at best and may be beyond the limits of the method: it may not be impossible but is at least questionable. How is the axis to be determined? On the basis of the whole complex or only the blocked portion? Amplitude or area? This problem is not addressed by all authors who discuss the subject, but is important.

If the patient is one in whom the diagnosis of left anterior hemiblock has been established, the addition of right bundle branch block in later tracings can be recognized easily, and the diagnosis of both is clearly justifiable, but this requires more than one tracing, and its prognostic value is still open to question. Several studies have failed to show that patients with right bundle branch block and left axis deviation (by various criteria) are significantly more likely to develop third-degree AV block than other members of the population.[518,522,526,548,647]

If the question of prophylactic pacing arises in a patient in the coronary care unit, the problem is not nearly so great. This patient probably has active heart disease in the first place, the facilities for pacing are immediately at hand, and the procedure involves only transient discomfort and little added expense, not commitment to permanent pacing. The elderly patient with right bundle branch block and left axis deviation who is to undergo surgery but has no clinical heart disease presents another special case. Here temporary pacing may be justified on the basis of its doing no harm and perhaps being life-saving, but prospective studies have indicated that even in this setting, the risk of the pacemaker is greater than its benefit.[548]

AV block may result from a combination of lesions distal to the bifurcation of the bundle of His,[136] and the typical pattern of IV block may result from local lesions above the bifurcation,[546] but it still is not possible to identify these without the aid of special intracardiac recording techniques.[101] *"Bilateral bundle branch block"* is a reasonable hypothesis but hard to prove.[144,177,178]

Miscellaneous Modifications of Intraventricular Conduction

The QRS complex may be prolonged and show notching and slurring throughout without producing the pattern of either right or left bundle branch block. This has been described under such headings as *arborization block*,[16] *parietal block*,[195] and *peri-infarction block*.[14,196-198] There never has been good agreement as to criteria for the diagnosis of peri-infarction block, and it seems more logical to diagnose myocardial infarction by the usual criteria and to make a separate diagnosis of IV conduction defect if necessary.

Sometimes QRS complexes of supraventricular origin, singly or in groups, are deformed in a manner implying change in the route of ventricular depolarization, *ventricular aberration*.[199-201,459,540,577] This is especially common with tachycardias originating in the atria but occurs also with isolated premature atrial contractions. The configuration of the QRS is usually similiar to that of right bundle branch block and presumably represents transient physiologic changes in conduction related to refractory periods and necessitating a different course of depolarization. The most important reason to recognize ventricular aberration is that, unrecognized, it might be interpreted as evidence of ventricular tachycardia.

Fusion beats are beats in which the QRS configuration represents depolarization of the ventricles from two sites at the same time, commonly a premature ventricular contraction and a normally conducted impulse, with a configuration not characteristic of either alone but with elements of both.[444]

Quinidine and similar drugs can deform the QRS by producing prolongation of the whole complex without change in configuration (see page 161). *Hyperkalemia* has the same general effect,[443,516] and these are almost the only nonstructural changes that modify the QRS significantly.

Summary and Clinical Comments

Block of either the right or the left branch of the bundle of His is the most common form of intraventricular conduction delay. It is recognized electrocardiographically by prolongation of the QRS complex to 0.12 sec or more with the terminal forces directed toward the block, i.e., broad, slurred terminal QRS deflections, positive in V_1 and usually negative in lead 1, with right bundle branch block, and positive in 1 and V_6 with left (in left bundle branch block the whole complex may be deformed, not just the terminal portion). The interpretation of certain EKG patterns as evidence of localized delay of intraventricular conduction, and the assumption that they imply a local lesion in a discrete subdivision of the left bundle branch, is a controversial hypothesis for which proof is not possible in the present state of things, even at autopsy. There is experimental, anatomic, and clinical evidence to support the idea, though, and it has useful clinical application; the presence of left or right bundle branch block is almost equally hard to prove, and these diagnoses are accepted universally. Delay, or block, of conduction in subdivisions of the left bundle branch may occur in any degree, in various combinations, and the lesion responsible may be in the parietal branches themselves or more proximal, even in the bundle of His. Intraventricular block has no clinical significance in itself and must be interpreted carefully in light of limitations indicated here, serial changes, and the clinical picture. The diagnosis implies a local lesion, structural or functional, and its significance is that of what caused it, often coronary atherosclerosis but sometimes trauma,[205] congenital,[206] idiopathic cardiac myopathy, or any other cause of myocardial disease. Left anterior hemiblock as an isolated finding is so common in elderly people that it usually has no immediate clinical impact and presumably reflects patchy fibrosis.

When block of the left bundle is proximal enough to distort initial QRS contour, it may obscure evidence of myocardial infarction, the diagnosis of which depends on findings in the first part of the complex, but left bundle branch block does not necessarily preclude a diagnosis of infarction. Pragmatically, myocardial infarction is a common cause of left bundle branch block. Each signifies scarring of the myocardium and if the criteria for both are fulfilled both may be diagnosed.[192,207,208,478] Right bundle branch block, manifest in the terminal part of the QRS complex, does not interfere with the diagnosis of infarction.

Bundle branch block and ventricular hypertrophy may coexist, and it is probable that the voltage criteria for hypertrophy are not changed significantly by block of either bundle branch.[209-211,442] The diagnosis of hypertrophy of the opposite ventricle in the presence of bundle branch block, however, is tenuous. The effect of the diagnosis of left bundle branch block of any other intraventricular conduction defect is to recognize that there is a local lesion in the myocardium, and this is in contrast to a diagnosis of hypertrophy with its implication of a hemodynamic burden.

Bundle branch block by itself does not produce serious hemodynamic changes,[450] but it may cause wide splitting of the first heart sound and, in the case of left bundle branch block, paradoxical splitting of the second one.

Bundle branch block is likely to be a fixed finding in serial electrocardiograms, but it may be intermittent[212,213] — found in some tracings and not in others or even in some beats and not others in the same tracing. It may be rate dependent, either fast or slow,[214-216,481,490,658] may be an apparently benign finding;[217,401] and may alternate between right and left.[659] It has been reported as hereditary[541] and has been found in healthy athletes.[525]

CHAPTER X

Structure and Function

The QRS complex can be seen as a reflection of ventricular anatomy — the ST-T-U, ventricular function. Structural change is manifest in the QRS while more subtle events affecting only function are recognized in the ST-T-U. The specificity-sensitivity spectrum of the ventricular complex can be compared to a pennant on a pole; a small breeze will be apparent only in the tip, a stronger one will straighten it out all the way, and a real hurricane will bend the pole; changes in the pennant alone will go away when the wind subsides, but those in the pole will not (Figure 10-1). T-wave abnormalities may result from almost any stimulus, ST-segment displacement requires a more severe or more sustained one, and (with few exceptions) QRS deformity implies structural change in the ventricular myocardium or its conduction system and is likely to be permanent. Structure and function are too closely related to be considered completely separately, but they are not the same, and the components of the EKG that reflect them must be described as precisely as possible before a value is assigned to each and its place in the diagnosis identified.

STRUCTURE

The *P wave*, written during atrial depolarization, represents atrial anatomy. Theoretically there is a T_a or P_t wave that represents atrial repolarization, but in practice this is not seen in the surface EKG. The atria have no thickness from an electrical point of view and a great deal less information can be obtained from a P than from a QRS. The whole atrial complex is called *P* whether it is positive,

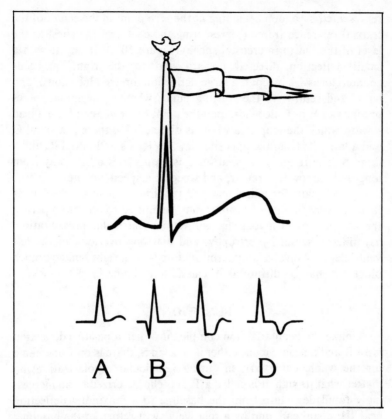

Figure 10-1. The QRS-T complex is more sensitive to the right and more specific to the left; the T wave is susceptible to many influences, the QRS to few. The tracing labeled A represents normal. In B there is abnormality of QRS implying structural change in the ventricular myocardium; in C, the ST segment is displaced, signifying injury; and in D abnormality is limited to the distal end of ST-T, the T wave, and is least specific of all.

negative or biphasic. Its characteristics have been described (see pages 47, 52).

Description of the *QRS* includes its orientation, duration, and, contour, and the first two of these have been discussed earlier (see pages 34, 47). The contour of the typical QRS can be described readily using vectorcardiographic terminology. Think of the QRS as represented by a loop beginning at the zero point in the center of the triaxial reference frame (representing the center of the chest at the level of the fourth intercostal space) (Figure 10-2). It begins with a small deflection directed upward and to the right, proceeds counterclockwise through a large deflection directed left, down, and back, and returns to the starting point; whether the initial forces produce an R or Q depends upon the point of view. Seen from a lead toward which the loop as a whole is directed, V_6, there is a small Q and a large R; from the opposite view, aVR, a small initial R, and a large S. The range of normal for this loop varies all the way from long and narrow to circular, and whether a specific complex is normal or not calls for judgement and requires consideration of other factors. Abnormality of contour may be limited to the initial part of the complex as in myocardial infarction ventricular preexcitation, asymmetric septal hypertrophy, and diastolic overload of the left ventricle, may involve only terminal forces as in right bundle branch block, or may be diffuse as in classic left bundle branch block.

FUNCTION

Unlike the depolarization complex in which a positive deflection is an R and a negative one either a Q or an S, there is only one name for the whole curve written during ventricular repolarization; no matter what its sign, it is called a T. It is characterized by an increasingly rapid departure from the baseline to a maximum deflection near the distal end, and by a relatively swift return to the baseline.

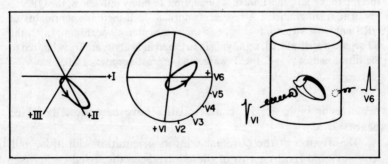

Figure 10-2. The QRS loop in space is characterized by a small initial deflection to the right, up, and forward followed by a large, smooth excursion to the left, down, and back ending with a return to the starting point.

Experience has taught that this curve can be divided into two components for analysis; a proximal, low frequency, basically horizontal one, the ST segment, and a distal, higher frequency, fundamentally vertical one, called T. This use of the same name for the complete curve and for one of its components leads to confusion, and when it is important to indicate that the whole complex is implied it must be called the ST-T.

The *T-wave* in a given lead is described under three headings: amplitude, sign, and a combination of these plus time, i.e., contour. *Amplitude* can be stated quantitatively and *sign* is either positive or negative, but *contour* must be described subjectively, and adjectives such as peaked, symmetrical, and rounded are used when it is abnormal.

The spatial orientation of T must be identified and its relation to that of QRS evaluated. Normally T is very close to QRS, the angle between them being no more than about 45° in the frontal plane and perhaps a little larger in the horizontal. Evaluation of this relationship is an important part of the analysis of every tracing, and the method has been described on pages 19, 34. In terms of the elephant-in-the-box analogy, it is comparable to determining whether the parts of the elephant are normal with relation to each other. A very wide spatial QRS-T angle is an abnormality that must be taken into account in the interpretation. In the normal subject, T is positive in leads taken from the left side of the chest and may be either positive or negative in those from the right.

The proximal part of the curve, the *ST segment*, is treated as a horizontal value, and abnormalities in it can be described by words that relate to horizontal things generally, displacement and contour. *Displacement* of ST is present when the J point, the *point* at which ST can be distinguished from QRS, is above or below the level of the PQ segment. The distance between these two levels is a measure of the strength of repolarization forces at the time the stylus becomes available for recording them after the larger ones generated during depolarization have been written. It is much more difficult to describe abnormalities of shape, or *contour*, of the *line* that follows J, the ST segment, than to measure displacement, but sagging, flattened and arched will serve satisfactorily in most instances.

The *U wave* is a low-frequency, low-amplitude deflection that may be of the same sign as the T or opposite and can be found in most tracings, commonly in right precordial leads. It need not be described routinely but must be noted when prominent. Sometimes, when it is of opposite sign from the T and continuous with it, it produces the illusion of terminal T abnormality; the two may be inseparable, and a very long "QT interval" will be measured. When the QT is found to be more than about 0.44 sec the chances are that a U is being included. The only way the U can be identified with confidence in such instances is to find a "dimple" where it merges with the T, and this is usually seen best in a right precordial lead.

CHAPTER XI

Abnormalities of Repolarization

ST-T abnormalities may be primary or secondary, i.e., they may reflect changes in the electrophysiology of repolarization in the absence of structural change, or they may follow abnormalities of structure that modify the route of depolarization without altering physiology (see Chapter III).

Abnormalities of T

Perhaps the most common abnormality to be found in electrocardiograms is lowering of T voltage, at least in frontal leads. Whether the voltage is truly low or low in a given lead or plane because it represents forces perpendicular to that lead or plane is a subject to be considered but not always to be resolved. Just how low a T must be to be called abnormal is a matter of judgment; it is evaluated in relation to QRS voltage, not an absolute set of figures, and a good criterion as an arbitrary starting point is that in a lead in which the QRS is almost completely positive and T is of the same sign (lead I or V_6, for instance), T amplitude should be at least 10% of that of QRS. Abnormalities of ST must be described separately, but when neither ST nor T findings, by themselves or in association with other abnormalities, fit into a pattern that points to a specific explanation for them, they are called *nonspecific ST-T abnormalities* (Figure 11-1).

Tracings showing only nonspecific findings must be interpreted very conservatively and with awareness of the patient's clinical problem. Almost anything can produce abnormalities of this sort (low T voltage, sagging/flattened ST); there may not be any heart disease at all. Such findings have been compared in their non-

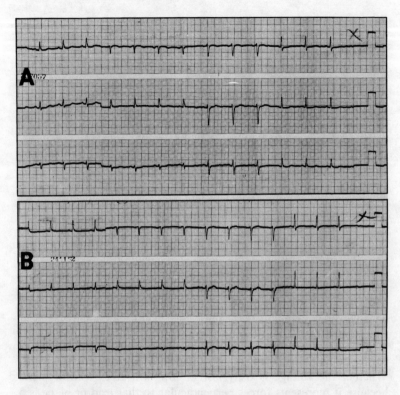

Figure 11-1. Nonspecific ST-T abnormalities. Low T voltage, especially in the frontal leads, is often associated with sagging/flattening of ST. The pattern is very common, not typical of anything, and can only be called a nonspecific abnormality. It does not always mean heart disease, and its clinical significance cannot be determined from the tracing alone.

specificity to elevation of the sedimentation rate,[19] but the sed rate is reported by a technician as a number, and ST-T abnormalities represent professional judgment. They are more like nausea and vomiting. Nausea and vomiting reflect events in the stomach, to be sure, but not always disease of the stomach; on the contrary, they often represent the response of a normal organ to stimuli arising elsewhere.

A classic way to bring about change experimentally in the T wave is to compromise the blood supply to the myocardium by ligating a coronary artery.[218,219] For this reason, as well as because a common basis for T-wave abnormalities in clinical experience is impairment of blood supply, T-wave abnormalities often seem to have been equated with ischemia, but this is an oversimplification of the problem. Remember, the EKG shows findings, results, but does not tell what produced them.

Discrepancy between the supply of blood and the demand for it may result from deficiency of supply, excess of demand, or both, and may be great or small. If great enough it causes infarction, mechanism disorder, or some other abnormality depending upon where it is. If very small, it may induce only minimal and non-specific changes in the tracing; intermediate degrees produce patterns that can be interpreted with varying degrees of confidence. When the discrepancy is the result of a *hemodynamic burden* as with left ventricular overload, the contour of T remains almost normal but its direction is away from the left ventricle, nearly opposite QRS, i.e., QRS is positive and T is negative in left chest leads (Figure 11-2A). (See page 128 for discussion of left ventricular strain.) When inadequacy is caused by impairment of blood supply, the location of the T abnormality depends upon the location of the lesion and may simulate the pattern of left ventricular overload almost precisely. The contour of T is more likely to be symmetrical when the problem is coronary artery disease than when it is left ventricular overload, but which mechanism, overload or undersupply, is responsible may not be apparent from a single tracing. When they are *transient* and associated with chest *pain*, these ST-T abnormalities are strong evidence for a diagnosis of coronary artery disease; when stable and accompanied by a more secure evidence of overload of the left ventricle, e.g., the high voltage of hypertrophy or a history of aortic valve disease, they may be assumed to be a result of left ventricular overload. When T is negative in midprecordial leads and deeper there than in V_1 or V_6, especially if very deep and symmetrical, the chances are that the underlying lesion is anterior *myocardial hypoxia* as with coronary atherosclerosis (Figure 11-2B). This pattern may correlate with localized hypertrophy,[697] and mechanisms of compromising oxygen delivery other than by stenosis of a coronary artery must be considered, e.g., anemia, shock. It is not unusual for left ventricular overload and coronary insufficiency to be present at the same time, and findings may be typical of both (Figure 11-2C).

When precordial T negativity cannot be explained by either left ventricular overload or impairment of blood supply, it is nonspecific and may be an unusual variant of normal;[14,222,466,553] negative precor-

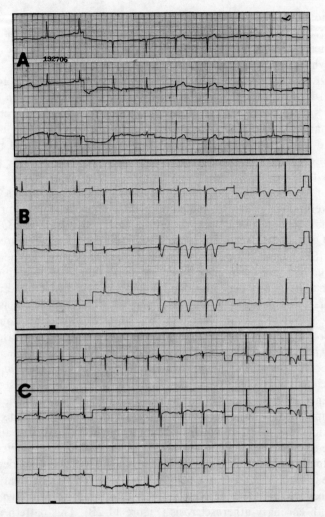

Figure 11-2. Left ventricular overload and coronary insufficiency. Abnormalities limited to T often reflect discrepancy between supply of blood to the myocardium and demand for it. When T is of normal contour and opposite QRS as in the top tracing, left ventricular overload, or "strain," is the most likely explanation; when symmetrical and deeper in midprecordial leads than in medial and lateral ones, coronary insufficiency (middle tracing). Both patterns may be seen in the same tracing (bottom). While these are typical and common, their overlap is wide, and the inherent nonspecificity of T abnormalities must be kept in mind.

dial Ts have been described in healthy young athletes,[554] and a very similar pattern has been reported as a result of pheochromocytoma,[643] in patients with hyperparathyroidism,[681] subarachnoid hemorrhage,[503] and concussion.[595] Tall, peaked precordial Ts are common in normals but may be one of the stigmata of hyperkalemia,[220,221] may reflect intracranial lesions,[362,364,365,595] and may have the same significance as deep, symmetric negativity, implying coronary insufficiency in a different vascular bed. Remember that the T wave, the distal end of the ST-T complex, is the most sensitive part of the tracing and that application of findings here requires the greatest clinical judgment.

An unusual finding, T alternans, alternation of T amplitude from beat to beat, is rare and of uncertain significance[471,545,671] (see page 165).

Mitral valve prolapse is often associated with negative T2,3,F, a pattern very similar to that of left ventricular overload but seen from below instead of from the left.[693]

Abnormalities of ST

The word *injury* is one of the rare examples in electrocardiographic jargon of a word from the common language used in exactly the same sense as in everyday life. It means not just damage but specifically damage to biologic structures — and transient damage at that. Injured tissue gets well or dies, and evidence of injury implies that the event that produced it happened recently. EKG evidence of myocardial injury is one of the most secure diagnoses that can be made and one of the easiest. ST displacement, when abnormal, means injury, the only exception being its persistence as evidence of a ventricular aneurysm.

An explanation for the changes of myocardial injury is suggested in Figure 11-3. From an electrophysiologic point of view, injury may be defined as inability of the damaged myocardium to repolarize completely though still capable of being depolarized. Figure 11-3A shows a resting muscle strip in a volume conductor with a unipolar electrode at each end, with each electrode connected to the positive pole of a galvanometer. This tissue is polarized, no potential difference is detectable in the volume conductor, and neither galvanometer shows any deflection; straight lines are written by the recorders. In Figure 11-3B the shaded area at the right represents injury. Because this tissue cannot be polarized completely and because the normal, unshaded portion of the strip *is* polarized, a boundary of potential difference exists between the two parts with injured portion less positive (i.e., negative) and a "current of injury" flows. The electrode at the left now faces the positive side of the boundary of potential difference (and difference in potential is what the EKG shows) and records a positive deflection, while that on the right faces the negative side of the boundary and its galvanometer indicates a negative quantity as evidence of the same abnormality, the "current of injury."

Figure 11-3C shows what happens when the strip is depolarized from left to right. The whole tissue is capable of depolarization and this produces an upstroke as viewed from the electrode toward which depolarization moves and a downstroke from the other, the process not being affected detectably by the injury. When the whole strip has been depolarized, there is no longer any difference of potential in the system and the trace returns to the baseline. In Figure 11-3D the boundary of potential difference due to injury is reestablished as the tissue is repolarized, the current of injury flows again, and the trace resumes the level that is a measure of the potential difference.

Figure 11-3E shows schematically how similar the foregoing examples are to the situation that exists when a layer of muscle beneath the epicardium of the left ventricle is injured. The electrode at the left of the figure may be compared to aVR and that at the right to V_6. The tracing shows ST displacement characteristic of superficial, *subepicardial*, injury, almost exactly a statement of the case in pericarditis (Figure 11-4A). The pericardium is not active electrically, but the myocardium immediately beneath it is, and the only route to this is through the epicardium. Subepicardial injury means pericardial inflammation but does not give any indication as to etiology. Figure 11-3F shows the situation reversed, i.e., deep or *subendocardial* injury a very common pattern. Theoretically, it could be produced by endocardial injury by means of a catheter, a pacemaker electrode, or a wayward central venous pressure line, but the nonlinear character of transmural sensitivity (see below) is such that the only way it really is produced is by impairment of blood supply; flattened depression of ST is typical of coronary insufficiency (Figure 11-4B). It is a more secure basis for the diagnosis than the T abnormality discussed above, but is often stable and asymptomatic in older people and not synonomous with angina.[672] This is a concept

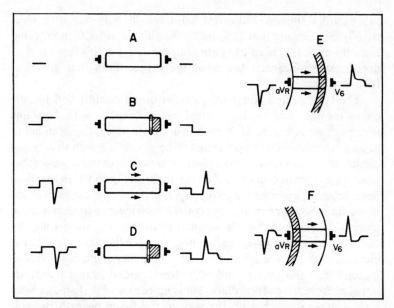

Figure 11-3. Derivation of ST displacement of injury. The muscle strip in A is resting, polarized, and no difference in potential is apparent. In B the right end of the strip has been injured, i.e., it is no longer completely polarized. This means that it is negative with relation to the rest of the strip and that a "current of injury" flows between the two. Seen from the right side, this difference in potential registers as a negative value; from the left, a positive one. In C the strip is depolarized from left to right and a QRS complex is generated. In D, repolarization has occurred and, the injured area not being capable of complete repolarization, the boundary of potential difference has been reestablished. The strips as indicated are comparable to a segment of the ventricular myocardium. In E the area of injury is beneath the epicardium and in F it is beneath the endocardium. The electrodes shown compare to aVR on the left and V6 on the right.

basic to understanding stress tests for coronary insufficiency (see page 149).

Clinical Significance of Injury Patterns

There are important differences, both qualitative and quantitative, between the significance of subendocardial injury and that of subepicardial injury. Subepicardial tissue is very sensitive electrically,[225] a feature that explains the usefulness of EKG monitoring from the exploring needle in pericardiocentesis, but this is not true of deeper, subendocardial layers of the myocardium that are electrically silent.[226-228]

The typical, and common, patterns of pericarditis and of coronary insufficiency are logical and easy to explain with diagrams such as those in Figure 11-3, but the direction of ST displacement in acute myocardial infarction seems to be in conflict with this. Myocardial infarction is subendocardial by nature, with the R wave (that must be present in order to define the abnormal Q on which the diagnosis is based) generated in tissue superficial to it. On the basis of the discussion above one might expect the ST segment to be depressed in anterior leads when there is an anterior infarct, but such is not the case; it may be depressed during angina preceding infarction but is elevated with the acute infarct itself. The injury implicit in ST displacement in this case is, indeed, subendocardial in that it extends outward from the endocardium, but is more extensive than seen with typical angina, reaches all the way to the tissue beneath the epicardium, and is reflected as subepicardial injury.[529,578,668] This same explanation may be relevant to the findings in Prinzmetal's, or "variant", angina, as may the possibility that the location of the lesion is simply on the opposite side of the heart from where one suspects it to be and from which conventional ST displacement would be recorded. The persistence of ST displacement characteristic of ventricular aneurysm (see page 121) also is unsatisfactorily explained, but identification of this depends upon serial tracings.

Definition of abnormality of ST displacement can be a vexing problem. In most tracings from normal hearts forces developed during repolarization are so small that by the time the stylus becomes available to record them (after depolarization has been completed) the trace is at substantially the same level as the baseline. In others, however, voltage at this juncture, the J point, is great enough that the trace is well away from the baseline on the way to writing the peak of the T wave. Elevation of ST with tall QRS and T in left chest leads may be seen as suggesting subepicardial injury, and in this setting the contour of ST assumes increased importance. If contour is normal, the pattern is within normal limits and is referred to for want of a better name as *"early repolarization"* (Figure 11-4C); when it is part of the T pattern of left ventricular overload, negative TV_{5-6}, the J

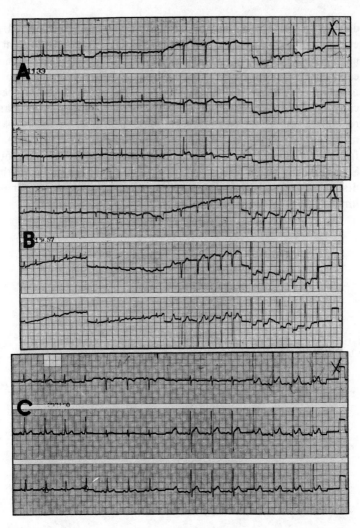

Figure 11-4. Myocardial injury. ST segment (J) displacement is almost synonymous with myocardial injury. When it is upward in precordial leads as in A above, it is typical of a subepicardial lesion; this, for practical purposes, means pericarditis but gives no indication of its etiology and must be differentiated from the normal "early repolarization" pattern in C, a decision that sometimes require serial tracings and awareness of the clinical setting. Subendocardial injury, as with coronary insufficiency, typically produces flattened depression of ST, B.

depression of "early repolarization" may be overinterpreted as evidence of coronary insufficiency. In the latter case, the patient is not likely to be hurt, but in the former, he may suffer at least unnecessary expense, anguish, and loss of time. A follow-up tracing hours or a day or two later will show changes if the pattern is due to pericarditis or coronary insufficiency and stability if it is that of "early repolarization."[510,512] In the normal electrocardiogram the ST segment is commonly a millimeter or more above the baseline in leads from the right side of the precordium but has a normal contour; ST contour is an important component of a decision as to whether displacement of the J point is or is not within normal limits.[223,224,510,512,669]

CHAPTER XII

Myocardial Infarction

There are two important sets of structural abnormalities that can be recognized from changes in depolarization — myocardial infarction and individual chamber enlargement — and three if intraventricular conduction defects (Chapter IX) are included.

The electrocardiographic diagnosis of infarction of the myocardium has three components: the lesion, its location, and its age. Recognition of the *lesion* itself depends upon abnormality of forces generated early in the course of ventricular depolarization as it proceeds from endocardium to epicardium — usually, but not always, an abnormal Q[229]. Processes other than infarction may produce exactly the same abnormalities, and it should be pointed out again that the EKG shows only the lesion, not what caused it.

The derivation of the abnormal Q of infarction is indicated in Figure 12-1. Consider two masses of muscle in a volume conductor depolarizing simultaneously in opposite directions and viewed from a single unipolar electrode placed so that the thicker mass depolarizes toward it and the thinner away from it. The result is as if a single force were directed toward the electrode, producing a positive deflection (Figure 12-1A). The shaded area in the second muscle strip represents dead tissue, tissue capable of transmitting the electricity but not of generating forces itself; the result is that at the beginning of depolarization the force directed away from the electrode is unopposed, the electrode sees the negative side of the boundary of potential difference, and a negative deflection is written. The late forces in this example are generated in the larger mass of muscle, after the process has been completed in the smaller one, and are directed to-

113

ward the electrode producing a final upstroke in the tracing (Figure 12-1B). Changes in the heart as a result of myocardial infarction are very similar to these, and a lead over the infarcted areas produces a view very similar to that of the exploring electrode in the example (Figure 12-1C).

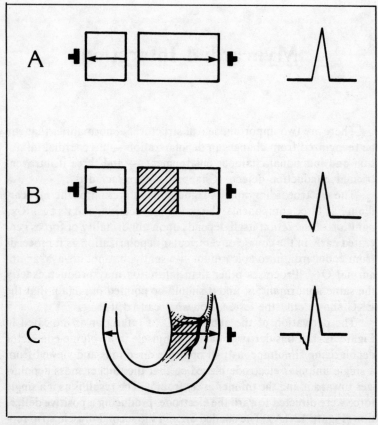

Figure 12-1. Origin of the pathologic Q wave of myocardial infarction. In A the small mass of muscle depolarizes to the left at the same time that the larger one depolarizes to the right, and the result is a net force to the right. In B the inner part of the large strip is dead, i.e., generates no voltage. Depolarization of the strip on the left away from the electrode is visible from the electrode as a negative deflection initiating events, but the final deflection is toward the electrode producing an upstroke. The similarity of the conditions in B to those in the wall of the left ventricle is suggested in C.

There are Q waves in nearly all electrocardiograms, the Q of infarction is an *abnormal* one, and the features that make it abnormal must be defined. A summary of what a Q is, and the characteristics of a normal one, will serve as a starting point. Consider the QRS loop (vectrocardiogram) in the frontal plane (See Figure 10-2). The small initial deflection, attributable to depolarization of the IV septum perceptibly before the mass of the ventricular wall, is an R when viewed from right and anterior leads (V_1 or V_2, and sometimes from aVR) and a Q from the left and posteriorly (I, aVL, V_6). Thus, leads with a tall QRS complex often have a small (not more than 0.03 sec in duration), clean, sharp Q, while those with a deep QRS are likely to begin with a tiny R.

There are two ways in which a Q wave may be abnormal: its *intrinsic* characteristics, contour and duration, and its *location*. A "dirty," wide Q, notched and irregular with a duration of 0.04 sec or more, is usually abnormal; depth is not an important criterion of abnormality. No matter how small and clean, a Q wave where a Q wave does not belong is abnormal and is strong evidence in favor of infarction. In normal precordial leads the first time an R wave is seen as one progresses from V_1 toward V_6, it will be initial. It will grow taller (relative to the S that follows it) in leads farther to the left (Figure 12-2) but may be preceded by a small clean Q in leads far to the left. As one goes from V_1 toward V_6 in the normal subject, a Q wave, once it appears, will be clean, sharp, and narrow, and will persist to the left and not grow smaller relative to the R that follows it. For instance, a clean, sharp QS is common in V_1 in normals and may be seen in V_2 or even farther to the left, but if there is an rSV_1 a QSV_2 is abnormal. A QSV_{1-2} followed by an rSV_3 is usually normal but a QSV_{1-2} followed by a $qrSV_3$ is not.

Recognition of abnormality of Q in inferior leads (2, 3, aVF) and lateral ones (I, L, V_6) depends almost entirely upon abnormalities of contour and duration and is much more difficult than in precordial leads. When there is clear ST-T evidence of injury, the diagnosis of any infarct is easier than when there is none.

Evidence of infarction may take forms other than a Q. A slurred, initial R in V_1 as a result of a dorsal infarct[230,231] is an example, and another is the early slurring or notching of a QS complex in right precordial leads with an anterior infarct.

The *localization* of an infarct is necessary for credibility of the di-

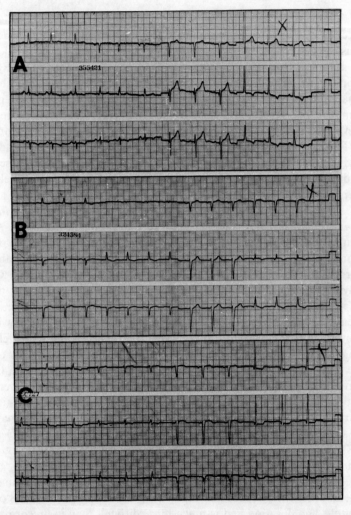

Figure 12-2. Anterior myocardial infarction. As one progresses from V₁ to V₆ in the normal tracing, the first time a positive deflection appears in the QRS, it should be initial and not grow smaller relative to its S in leads farther to the left. In leads from the left side of the chest where R is dominant, though, there may be a normal small Q. Once Q appears it does not grow smaller to the left. All three of the tracings here show old anterior infarcts. There is good evidence of left ventricular hypertrophy and strain also in A, there may be old inferior scarring as well as anterior in C, and in B the ST-T pattern suggests left ventricular overload.

agnosis but is of little importance in establishing prognosis.* The terminology in everyday use sometimes implies precision beyond the limits of the method; "anteroseptal," for instance, is used loosely in the literature, apparently synonymously with anteromedial, to indicate that the abnormality is seen in right precordial leads as distinguished from left. There is evidence that abnormalities here really mean involvement of the interventricular septum,[6,7] but this adds little. It is enough to designate the location of an infarct by telling where it is seen, i.e., *anterior* for one seen in precordial leads, *lateral* for one seen from the left side (leads I, L, and V6), and *inferior* when seen from below (leads 2, 3, and F) (Figure 12-3). A truly *dorsal* infact would be expected to enhance representation of forces directed anteriorly, producing an abnormal initial R in V1. This possibility must be borne in mind when dealing with atypical anterior forces, but anatomic correlation of findings in the electrocardiogram with isolated dorsal infarction has not been published yet. The differential diagnosis of abnormally directed anterior forces includes, in addition to dorsal infarction, right ventricular enlargement, right bundle branch block, anterior septal fascicular block,[580] and unusual patterns such as seen with Ebstein's anomaly of the tricuspid valve. Infarcts, of course, are not bounded by straight lines and may be seen from more than one view, e.g., anterolateral and inferodorsal.

Patterns have been proposed for recognition of infarction of papillary muscles[64] but are not generally accepted.[265] Infarction of only the deep layers of the myocardium, *subendocardial* infarction, must occur, but the electrocardiographic diagnosis of it as such probably is not possible.[266-270,405,674-676] There is impressive evidence that the inner layers of the myocardium are electrocardiographically inactive,[228] but the subject is still controversial.[227] Some authors distinguish between subendocardial and transmural infarction without making it clear how the distinction is made. One gets the impression from the literature that often an infarct is assumed to be limited to the subendocardial area when it is documented by means other than the electrocardiogram, especially if there is flattened ST depression

---

*An exception is that complete AV block is seen less frequently with anterior infarcts than with inferior ones but has a worse prognosis. It occurs in about 2% of anterior infarcts with a mortality on the order of 80% or greater as compared to about 8% of inferior ones with a mortality rate of 25%.[145,146,271]

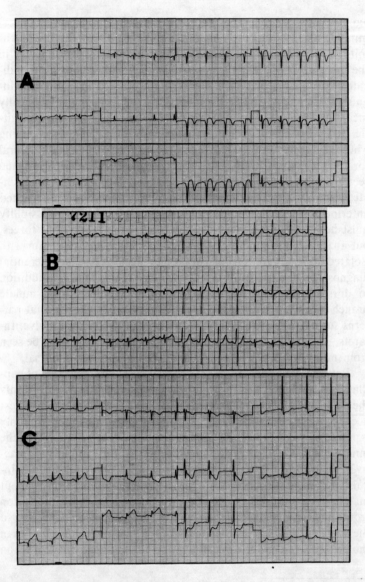

Figure 12-3. Acute myocardial infarction. In addition to deformity of the initial part of the QRS signifying a physical lesion, there is ST displacement typical of injury with its implication that something has happened recently. The aspect of the chest from which the findings can be seen best is stated also: A anterior, B lateral, and C inferior.

in precordial leads; transmural if there is a typical QR pattern. To suspect a subendocardial infarct on the basis of these criteria is logical, but proof that such is the case is not clear, and to call an infarct transmural when it presents as a QR is not logical at all, since the R in the QR pattern must derive from tissue superficial to the infarct. Transmural infarction produces a QS pattern in a lead taken from over its surface.[323] Infarction, or scarring, that is entirely intramural may be recognized but requires special techniques.[5,226,673]

Illogical though it may be, sometimes it is possible to make a diagnosis of myocardial infarction, or at least to suspect it, from a QR configuration of a premature ventricular contraction.[272-274]

A statement as to the *age of the lesion* is necessary. Whether it is old or new is judged from the presence or absence of ST displacement; (i.e., injury), the assumption being that injury, if present, is part of the same lesion that produced the infarct. Injury is a self-limiting thing; it does not last forever, the tissue either dies or recovers. If there is ST displacement in the presence of QRS evidence of infarction, the lesion is assumed to be of recent origin. Such ST displacement usually lasts no more than three or four weeks and often very much less, sometimes minutes or hours, and sometimes it may not be seen at all. Another basis for calling an infarct recent is to find evidence of it in a current tracing that had not been in one made a short time before. Truly transmural infarcts produce little ST displacement.[232] Absence of ST-T findings typical of injury justifies the assumption that the lesion is old — but does not prove that it is.

In summary, the common and confident EKG diagnosis of myocardial infarction rests on several assumptions. Having diagnosed a structural lesion in the presence of injury, we assume that both are due to the same thing and that, whatever that is, it must have occurred recently. Next, we judge that the most likely basis for all this is infarction — and of course we are usually right. A rare but sometimes important exception to this logic is the persistent ST displacement of a ventricular aneurysm, and this is not a very dangerous problem since there is an infarct in these cases though it is not new.

Accuracy of the Electrocardiogram in Myocardial Infarction

Published studies of the value of the electrocardiogram in making the diagnosis of myocardial infarction[233-235,441] agree that accuracy is considerable if the infarct is recent, probably above 90%, but much less when the lesion is old, as low as 25%. Quantitative criteria for definition of infarction at autopsy, techniques of dissection, and electrocardiographic standards all vary, and absolute figures cannot be had. Clinical experience teaches if the EKG abnormalities typical of recent infarction are present, the diagnosis will be accurate in nearly all cases, and good evidence of an old infarct is almost as dependable. From the opposite point of view, though, it must be realized that even a new infarct, much less an old one, may be present without there being diagnostic changes in the tracing. In the case of a recent one there will be at least nonspecific abnormalities in almost 100% of the cases, but with an old one the tracing may be normal.[236-239] To summarize, a well-founded electrocardiographic diagnosis of myocardial infarction is almost certain to be correct, but absence of evidence is not evidence of absence. Stigmata of an infarct may be cancelled by a second one,[644,676] or by coronary artery bypass grafts,[626-627] and an old one may leave no residual abnormality at all. To "rule out" an infarct is like trying to "rule out" flying saucers; it cannot be done. A normal tracing practically excludes the diagnosis of a *recent* infarct but not the presence of extensive coronary atherosclerosis.[240]

Differential Diagnosis of EKG Evidence of Myocardial Infarction

If one recognizes that the etiology of abnormalities in the electrocardiogram is not implicit in them, that the findings we label infarction would be identified better as evidence of a lesion, the possibilities for false positives become obvious. There may be false negatives, too, and infarction may occur without recognizable clinical symptoms.[625] Failure to recognize an infarct from the tracing when one is present is not very likely to hurt the patient because there are other means of identifying infarcts, but a diagnosis of an infarct when one is not present, a false positive, is one of the insidious dangers of the method; once the diagnosis has been made, there is no way to remove it completely, no way to "rule out" an infarct with absolute confidence.

Mechanisms by which false positives (and sometimes false negatives) may be produced are several. First, of course, the *limits of the method*; normal findings overlap abnormal to a considerable degree. It is not just a Q wave that is the usual sign of infarction but an abnormal Q, and definition of abnormal is not precise. Qs that could easily be called abnormal are found sometimes even in healthy young people.[258,259] Pectus excavatum is often associated with prominent Q's.[242,243,613] EKG changes due to hyperkalemia may simulate infarction,[249,516,664] and so may other *noncardiac diseases*, e.g., pulmonary disease, especially embolism or cor pulmonale[614] (see page 164), pancreatitis,[241] penumothorax,[251,493,615] and blunt trauma[252,616] (see page 166). Precordial Q waves may be rate dependent.[665]

Diseases of the heart other than infarction explain many false positives. Not many congential lesions present the problem, but corrected transposition and subendocardial fibroelastosis have been reported to produce false positives.[247,629] Ventricular preexcitation (as with the Wolff-Parkinson-White syndrome) is a common offender,[189,191,618] and scarring may be part of idiopathic cardiac myopathy,[244-246] sarcoid,[619] amyloid, muscular dystrophy,[620] or infectious mononucleosis.[617] Asymmetric septal hypertrophy[452] may change the initial part of the QRS as a result of enlarging the mass of the IV septum, and left ventricular hypertrophy alone may do the same thing.[256,257,452] Left anterior hemiblock has been reported as mimicking myocardial infarction,[440,511,538,621,622,691] as has mitral valve prolapse,[502] and focal block of septal ramifications of the left bundle has been proposed as still another explanation for abnormal Q waves.[699] Dorsal infarction may be stimulated by abnormally directed anterior forces resulting from block of a septal segment of the intraventricular conduction system.[623] Right atrial enlargement may be a big factor in abnormality of the Q[248], pericardial effusion has been found as the explanation for EKG findings of infarction,[624] and false positives due to cardiac surgery[250] are easy to understand. Similar findings may be produced on occasion by artificial ventricular pacemakers,[482,677] and distortion of the first part of the QRS by merging of P and QRS in isorhythmic dissociation has been seen.

Technical error can produce EKG findings that mimic myocardial infarction, most commonly transposition of left arm and leg leads, right arm and leg leads, occasionally right and left arm leads, and misplacement of the electrodes for precordial leads, e.g., transposition of V_1 and V_3. Individual leads mounted upside down can produce a problem. There are other circumstances in which one risks a false-positive diagnosis of infarction,[253-255] and anyone interpreting eletrocardiograms must be aware of the danger to the patient of such possibilities.

Infarcts may occur without clinical evidence,[625] so-called silent infarcts, and electrical evidence of death may precede structural death and be transient.[260-263] Evidence of infarction often disappears during follow-up of lesions that were well documented when acute, and it has been noted also that evidence may disappear following coronary artery bypass.[626,627]

False negatives are much less common and less likely to be a clinical problem. Third-degree AV block with idioventricular or artificial ventricular pacemaker, ventricular preexcitation, left bundle branch block, left anterior hemiblock,[628] and errors of lead placement, especially swapping of the left arm and leg leads, may obscure EKG evidence of infarction.

Miscellaneous

The *time* necessary for appearance of EKG exchanges in infarction is hard to specify. How long does it take for anatomic changes that can be recognized at autopsy to develop? How does one know when the infarct occurred? ST-T changes can appear almost immediately after compromise of blood supply, but observations following accidental occlusion of coronary arteries at surgery or coronary arteriography have led to the impression that the QRS changes of infarction may be delayed for as long as eight hours, and there is some evidence to support this.[413]

The *number* of myocardial infarcts that may be diagnosed from a *single* tracing is not greater than one. Infarction may be recognized from more than one view, anterior and inferior for instance, but on the basis of only one tracing one cannot be sure that this represents two lesions. With serial tracings two lesions (anterior and inferior) may be diagnosed, and perhaps a third (left lateral), but beyond this, evidence other than that from the electrocardiogram is needed for the diagnosis of multiple infarcts.[275]

The *complications* of myocardial infarction that are of electrocardiographic significance are mostly disorders of impulse formation and conduction, "electrical failure."[145,276-278] Persistence of ST displacement past the usual few days following an acute infarct is empirical evidence suggesting a *ventricular aneurysm*.[223,279,414]

Infarction of the *atrial* myocardium is recognized very rarely but does occur.[280-282,395,645]

CHAPTER XIII

Chamber Imbalance

The earliest clinical usefulness of electrocardiography was in the study of impulse formation and conduction and it remains the best method available for this purpose, but evaluation of coronary blood flow in patients with chest pain, and especially in the diagnosis of myocardial infarction, is probably its best known application. Less useful than either of these but still of importance is its potential value in pointing to one or more of the chambers of the heart as laboring under a disproportionate hemodynamic burden.

Atrial Enlargement

Overwork of one or both atria often can be inferred from the size and shape of P, but the range of normal is broad. Generally, *right atrial enlargement* ("P pulmonale") is suspected when the P wave is prominent (tall and peaked — both terms are relative) in leads 2, 3, and F[285,286] (Figure 13-1A); prominence of QV_1 may be evidence of right atrial enlargement, too.[248] *Left atrial enlargement* ("P mitrale") is recognized best by prominent terminal negativity of PV_1, i.e., its area is greater than 1 square millimeter[287-290] (Figure 13-1B); exaggerated notching of P, especially in lead 2, is common, but a small notch is not abnormal. The Marcruz index, the ratio of the duration of the P wave to that of the PR segment, has been proposed as a means of recognizing atrial enlargement but is not useful.[291]

Enlargement of an atrium may result from overload by either flow or resistance. Left atrial enlargement represents response to mitral regurgitation or stenosis or loss of compliance of the left ventricle; right, the same sort of abnormalities of the tricuspid valve and right ventricle. It may be transient, changing within hours in re-

123

sponse to treatment or even minutes as with exercise testing, and is probably related more to dilatation than to hypertrophy.

Ventricular Enlargement

On the basis of what we know about electrophysiology and anatomy, it would be logical to expect than an increase in myocardial mass (hypertrophy) of one ventricle out of proportion to the other would produce changes in the QRS — its orientation, duration (the time required for depolarization), and amplitude (the

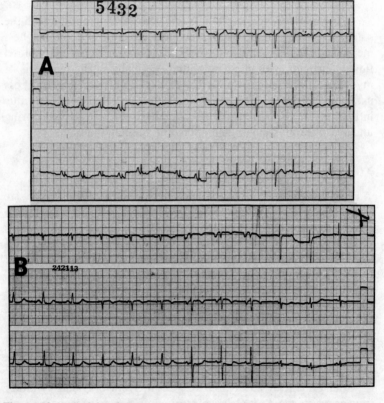

Figure 13-1. Atrial enlargement. Right atrial enlargement (A) increases forces directed downward and is apparent as prominent P2,3,F; left atrial enlargement (B), late P forces directed toward the back and producing prominent terminal negativity of PV₁.

voltage generated). If an appropriate increase in blood supply accompanied the hypertrophy, and no metabolic abnormalities occurred, no ST-T changes would be expected, but if the ventricle were to be loaded beyond its capacity, "strained," ST-T changes would be expected and it would be reasonable to predict that they would occur in a more or less consistent pattern in some manner suggestive of their origin. These hypotheses are logical, have a good basis in experimental and clinical observations, and can be applied effectively. They work.

Activation time. The time required for inscription of the QRS is independent of its amplitude; the greater the distance covered by the boundary of potential difference as it passes from endocardium to epicardium the longer the time it takes. In the example shown (Figure 13-2), the time required for depolarization is measured from the point at which the upstroke begins to the point at which it ends. The downstroke is the "intrinsic deflection," the deflection that occurs when the tissue intrinsic beneath the electrode is depolarized, and in this hypothetical example it is vertical. This concept is simplistic but makes some sense and has been transferred to the clinical electrocardiography. The idea is that a disproportionate increase in

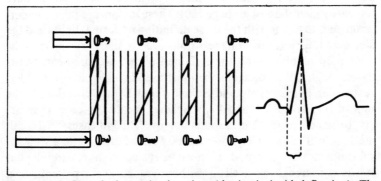

Figure 13-2. Ventricular activation time (the intrinsicoid deflection). The muscle strips on the left are being depolarized toward the electrodes. Note that the amplitude of the deflection varies inversely with the distance of the electrode from the potential it reflects but that its duration remains the same. The figure on the right indicates the duration of the time of onset of the intrinsicoid deflection, the ventricular activation time. This is a controversial concept and is rarely applied directly.

the thickness of the wall of one ventricle will require a longer time for that wall to be depolarized so that the upstroke in a lead whose positive electrode faces that ventricle will have a greater duration than normal. Because there are forces working in other directions at the same time, though, the intrinsic deflection is not vertical in the electrocardiogram and the downstroke of the QRS is called "intrinsicoid." Its *time* of onset is measured from the beginning of the QRS complex to the point where a perpendicular from the last positive peak intersects the baseline. In the normal adult, the time of onset of the intrinsicoid deflection, or *ventricular activation time,* in a left ventricular lead (one whose positive electrode faces the left ventricle) is not more than about 0.04 sec; in right ventricular leads (V_1 or V_2), 0.02 sec. The problem with this concept is that it is impractical in clinical application — one cannot interpret time intervals this closely in a routine tracing; it is not very helpful.

QRS amplitude. Though its value is limited by the wide range of normal, voltage has been shown by many investigators to be the most useful indicator of hypertrophy, especially when it is the left ventricle that is hypertrophied. The determinants of voltage are many in addition to the mass of ventricular muscle and its thickness. They include the distance of the electrode from the heart, the conductivity of intervening tissues, the volume and temperature of blood in the ventricle, the recording equipment, and others that are less easily identifiable (see page 160). These factors are poorly understood and, together with the loose definition of normal limits and the fact that the range of voltage within even a short tracing may be wide, they inhibit severely the usefulness of this measurement. Nonetheless, high QRS voltage is the most useful single indicator of left ventricular hypertrophy, and Sokolow and Lyon's criterion,[293] the sum of SV_1 and RV_5 (or RV_6, whichever is taller) greater than 3.5 mv, points correctly to it in something over 80% of cases.[294] To call the sum of SV_1 and RV_5 closer than 0.5 is not useful, and a value of 4.0 is not clearly abnormal; 4.5 must be evaluated more carefully but still is not enough by itself — without regard to the patient's age, habitus, and other clinical data — to make a diagnosis of left ventricular hypertrophy. At 5.0 mv left ventricular hypertrophy must be considered likely and dealt with in the diagnosis.

Right ventricular hypertrophy can be diagnosed with confidence when the QRS is directed straight forward and a little to the right, when $QRSV_1$ is predominantly positive and a prominent S wave persists as far left as V6, but patterns less clear-cut than this may be normal or reflect dilatation of the ventricle, and figures for QRS amplitude are not very useful.[295,296]

Spatial orientation of the QRS. Depolarization of a large mass of muscle generates a greater voltage and produces a larger deflection than depolarization of a small mass; hypertrophy of one ventricle, not balanced by equal hypertrophy of the other, would be expected to produce displacement of the net, or mean, QRS value proportionately — leftward, upward, and posteriorly in the case of the left ventricle, and rightward and anteriorly in the case of the right (Figure 13-3). These observations are logical but do not always work. "Axis deviation" may or may not occur and is not a reliable criterion for ventricular hypertrophy; when it does occur, it may represent left anterior (or posterior) hemiblock as a result of patchy fibrosis associated with hypertrophy rather than be a reflection of an increase in muscle mass.

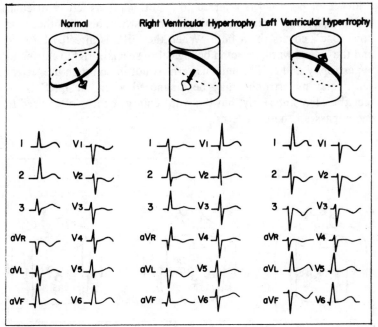

Figure 13-3. Diagramatic representation of mean spatial QRS in ventricular hypertrophy.

ST-T changes. When a ventricle is stressed beyond its comfortable capacity, it may be said to be strained. Circumstances producing such overload, abnormalities of either flow or resistance, result in changes of transmyocardial gradients of pressure and blood flow that alter the ST-T complex before anatomic change is manifest in the QRS. When there is discrepancy between blood flow and need for blood, the first part of the myocardium to suffer is the subendocardial region, and whether the discrepancy is the result of diminution of blood supply or increase in demand or both makes little difference in its manifestation in the tracing. The ST-T picture of left ventricular overload can be described succinctly as characterized by a QRS that points to the left and usually back and upward while the normally contoured T is directed almost opposite, i.e., there is a positive QRS in V6 with a negative T (Figure 13-4). J may be depressed, but in typical left ventricular overload ST is not flattened, and the J depression probably represents "early repolarization." The combination of QRS evidence of hypertrophy and ST-T evidence of overload is referred to traditionally as left ventricular hypertrophy and strain, but either may exist without the other, and "overload" covers them both. When the QRS is directed forward and the T backward, it would be logical to speak of right ventricular hypertrophy and strain, but this term is not in common use. Right ventricular hypertrophy may be diagnosed when the QRS is directed clearly anteriorly, but the word enlargement is often used to encompass all these patterns.

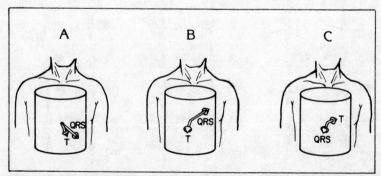

Figure 13-4. Ventricular strain. Strain (overload) of a ventricle is manifest by direction of T away from that ventricle, a sign that often appears before QRS evidence of increase in muscle mass, i.e., hypertrophy.

Discussion

It seems reasonable that it should be possible to recognize the early, physiologic manifestations of strain of a ventricle before the later, structural ones of hypertrophy have occurred; similarly, hypertrophy without strain might be expected in hearts in which increase in blood supply in response to overload has been adequate. Such patterns do occur but their specificity is limited. The one typical of strain involves only the T and the same abnormality can be produced from the other end of the physiologic system by restriction of coronary blood supply. Given serial tracings to establish the transient nature of the findings or their persistence, this "insufficiency pattern" can indeed be useful, at least as corroborative evidence when the clinical setting is known, but by itself in a single tracing it does little to distinguish between coronary artery disease and hemodynamic burden on the ventricle. Evidence of hypertrophy is a more dependable indicator of load on the ventricle but is not always conclusive.

The word hypertrophy means the same in electrocardiography as in any other muscle system, i.e., bigger, not just big but bigger, bigger than it was or than it should be by some arbitrary standard.* Hypoxia may be a factor in its pathogenesis,[570] but the basic stimulus to hypertrophy of any muscle is for it to be called upon to respond to a load beyond that which it can accomodate comfortably, i.e., strain or overload. A diagnosis of hypertrophy (based on findings in QRS) is more secure than one of strain (based on abnormality of T), but even when criteria for both are present there is room for error. The usefulness of both terms, hypertrophy and strain, is limited by two problems: first, they have been used so loosely and so long by so many that distinction between them has been blurred. Radiologists have not helped by referring to the x-ray picture of hypertrophy when what they see is mostly increase in volume. Enlargement is a less specific word, implying increase in either volume (dilatation) and/or mass (hypertrophy), and the diagnosis of left ventricular enlargement or left ventricular overload serves the purpose of directing attention to the left ventricle without implying a degree of specificity beyond the limits of the method.

---

*Hyperplasia has been shown to occur in the newborn,[547] but this is not of importance in adults.

The second limitation is that neither hypertrophy nor strain can be proved to exist. Despite the ease with which it can be defined qualitatively and the logical assumption that it would be identifiable at autopsy, quantitative criteria for definition of hypertrophy vary widely and there is much overlap between normal and abnormal. Echocardiography has been applied to this problem recently but so far has not had a major impact.[605] The concept of strain is clear, and most would not balk at some laboratory definition involving oxygen debt, lactic acid accumulation, frayed myofibrils, extravasation of red cells, etc., but apparently there have been no attempts to relate EKG findings to objective evidence of this sort.

How, then, is the diagnosis to be evaluated? With what can EKG findings be correlated so as to validate them? The most specific thing that can be identified in the series of events and their consequences that lead to selective overload of a ventricle is the presence or absence of a basis for it, i.e., overload. This has the advantage of being simple, easy, not requiring autopsy, and of being what we are really interested in anyway.

Overload of the *left ventricle* is, for practical purposes, a consequence of either one or both of only two possibilities; increase in flow (preload) and increase in resistance to output (afterload). Abnormalities of flow that overload the left ventricle (and not the right) are valve regurgitation (aortic and mitral) and shunts (ventricular septal defect and ductus arteriosus); increase in resistance may reside in the peripheral arterioles (hypertension), larger arteries (arteriosclerosis), aorta (coarctation), and/or left ventricular outflow obstruction (supravalvular, valvular, or subvalvular). That is all, and each of these can be identified easily by physical examination. Increase in resistance due to increase in blood viscosity would affect both ventricles.

In summary, if the sum of the amplitude of SV_1 and RV_5 (or RV_6, whichever is taller) is large, in the absence of another explanation for high voltage, left ventricular hypertrophy must be suspected; if the QRS is directed left, up, and back while the T is directed nearly opposite, overload, or strain (Figure 13-5) should be suspected, even though hypertrophy cannot be identified. Often both hypertrophy and strain are clear.

There are two classic patterns suggesting overload of the *right ventricle* (Figure 13-6), that due to an increase in resistance to outflow — systolic overload or "afterload," seen typically with pul-

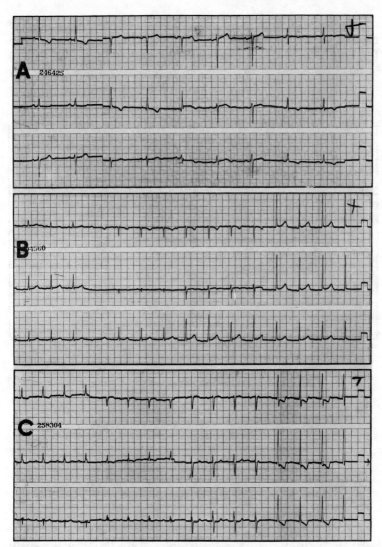

Figure 13-5. Left ventricular overload. Distinction between the ST-T change produced by overload, or strain, of the ventricle and QRS evidence of hypertrophy, a logical consequence of overload, is easy; the latter is the more secure diagnosis. Neither is likely to be of critical importance, and dilatation cannot be identified from the EKG. A, left ventricular strain without hypertrophy; B, left ventricular hypertrophy without strain; and C, left ventricular hypertrophy and strain.

monary stenosis; and that resulting from an increase in flow during diastole — diastolic overload or "preload," probably resulting more from dilatation than from hypertrophy and seen typically with an atrial septal defect.[403] In the first there is a qRV₁ with negative TV₁ and a prominent S in left precordial leads; in the latter, biphasic

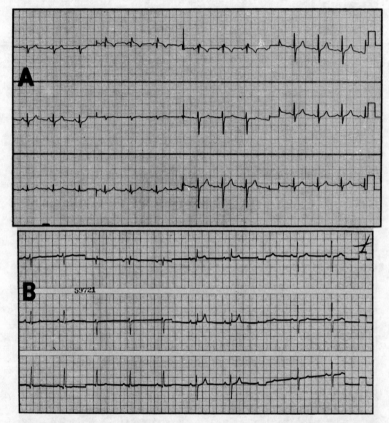

Figure 13-6. Right ventricular enlargement. When the QRS is directed anteriorly (B), especially if it is also to the right, a diagnosis of increased thickness of the right ventricular wall (hypertrophy) is usually justified. Often, though, biphasicity of QRS from all views is the consequence of right ventricular overload. This latter pattern (A) may be transient in association with events that produce acute hemodynamic burden on the right ventricle and may represent dilatation more than hypertrophy; it is often called enlargement.

QRS complex (S1,2,3) is present in almost all leads and often rSr in V₁. The first is clear evidence of hypertrophy, while the other may reflect dilatation and should be called enlargement. These patterns are not absolute by any means but are part of a continuum, merging with right bundle branch block and with normal, and distinction among them is not always possible. An unusual pattern that has been suggested as evidence of right ventricular overload is a "dome and dart" configuration the ST-T.[402]

The electrocardiographic definition of *biventricular hypertrophy* is a tenuous thing indeed. Little logic seems to be involved. Equal hypertrophy of both ventricles would be expected to result in either large complexes or no change in the electrocardiogram at all, and it is unlikely that hypertrophy of one ventricle or the other is ever completely isolated; there is no clear anatomic dividing line between the myocardium of the two and metabolic changes affecting either almost certainly affect both to some extent. Nonetheless, clinical experience leaves one with the clear impression that when the picture of left ventricular overload can be seen inferiorly (leads 2, 3 and F) better than laterally and coexists with evidence of right ventricular hypertrophy, one is justified in suspecting hypertrophy of both ventricles.[298]

Ventricular Hypertrophy and Bundle Branch Block

The diagnosis of bundle branch block depends upon QRS contour, while that of hypertrophy is based on voltage, and the two are not mutually exclusive. Each serves to direct attention to one ventricle or the other, but hypertrophy / strain / enlargement / overload imply a response to a hemodynamic load, while bundle branch block identifies the location of a lesion and requires a different line of investigation for its elucidation. Oftentimes distinction between the patterns of hypertrophy and bundle branch block is arbitrary.[299-301,442]

In summary, the diagnosis of ventricular overload, by whatever name, should have only one specific effect, to insure that the doctor considers the possibility of a hemodynamic burden seen by that ventricle so that he may determine whether one of the lesions that can produce it is present. Quantitative criteria for its recognition, and the terminology by which it is expressed, vary widely and the doctor who interprets the electrocardiogram, or the report of an electrocardiogram, must recognize the limitations of the method and the potential for harm to his patient. Ventricular hypertrophy is not a disease, and failure to recognize it from the tracing is not likely to hurt a patient who has had a history and physical examination, but its diagnosis may produce much harm if the physician does not appreciate the limitations of the method.

CHAPTER XIV

Methods

Many electrocardiographic abnormalities typical of disease can be simulated very closely by technical errors of recording, mounting, or labeling, and an important responsibility of the one who interprets the tracing is to identify these, correct for them when possible, and recognize the limitations they introduce when correction is not possible. The technician can be forgiven for making a mistake, but the doctor must not let the mistake work to the patient's detriment, and the best way to avoid this is for him not only to be aware of the problem but also to have had experience in recording and processing tracings and to understand the equipment involved.[375-379]

RECORDING THE TRACING

Preparation of the Patient

Skeletal muscle activity produces electrical currents and must be kept at a minimum during recording; the patient should be as relaxed as possible, and this is accomplished best by having him lie supine on a surface wide enough to support him comfortably. If this is not practical, there is no reason that a tracing cannot be made while the subject is seated, or in any other position, as long as this is noted. A few words of explanation and reassurance will help to control muscle tremor by lessening the fear and anxiety common in patients having an electrocardiogram made, especially their first one.

Attaching the Electrodes

With the machine turned on and ready to go, the electrode sites are prepared, and the electrodes are attached. The purpose of electrode jelly is to minimize skin resistance and provide good electrical contact with the recording equipment. The value of this step is less now than it was when recording depended more on the sensitivity of the system and less on amplification, but it is still important. The amount of jelly used should be just enough to moisten an area of skin the size of the electrode; too much not only makes a mess but also may introduce artifact. The jelly should be rubbed into the skin with some vigor — the edge of an electrode is a good instrument for this purpose. It is especially important in the precordial leads not to use too much because electrode positions here are close together, and if the area prepared for one position overlaps that for the next the result may be almost the same as if one big electrode covered both areas.[501]

Limb electrodes may be attached anywhere on a limb, since arms and legs act as linear conductors connected to the trunk at the shoulders and the symphysis pubis. If suction electrodes are used, those for the arms may be attached to the anterior aspect of the shoulders; if flat electrodes are held on by straps, it is best to apply them over soft tissues to insure good contact with their whole surface, high on the volar aspect of the forearms and the inner aspect of the calves are the usual places. The straps should be just tight enough to hold the electrodes on comfortably; if they are tight enough to cause discomfort or loose enough to allow the electrodes to slip, artifacts (wandering baseline or muscle tremor) may result. Tension on electrodes can be kept to a minimum by having the binding posts of those on the legs directed upward and those on the arms directed downward. If it is necessary to record a tracing from a patient one or more of whose extremities are missing or swathed in bandages, remember that electrodes can be attached to the stumps of limbs or directly to the body at the shoulders and symphysis pubis, and either or both of the leg electrodes can be attached to either leg, since both are effectively in continuity with the body at the inferior angle of Einthoven's triangle — the symphysis pubis. When the chest is bandaged or for some other reason it is not possible to place precordial electrodes in their standard positions, tracings may be recorded from other points but the location of these must be understood by the interpreter.

Grounding the Equipment

In order for the small electrical potentials generated in the heart to be seen, other signals must be eliminated. The most troublesome source of unwanted electrical activity is alternating current. Alternating current, AC (as distinct from direct current or DC), reverses its polarity (alternates) 60 times a second, broadcasting an electromagnetic field in its vicinity, and both the patient and the EKG machine act as antennae to receive this signal. The EKG machine (the galvanometer) must be attached to an external AC power supply (unless battery operated), and the patient-machine system and the power supply itself comprise a single functional unit all of which must be kept at the same electrical level. If they are not, if there are differences of potential within the system, the galvanometer indicates these as well as the ones that arise in the heart. In order to prevent 60-cycle interference, all components of the system must have the same potential-to-ground. This is assured by connecting the frame of the machine to the earth itself on one side via the power supply and to the patient on the other via the right leg lead. Thus, when properly connected, the patient is in electrical continuity with the EKG machine, which is grounded. There is no difference in potential-to-ground between any two parts of the system, and the galvanometer shows only the electrical events within the system itself, i.e., those occurring in the heart.

If this system is modified by the patient's being in contact with other electrical equipment with a potential-to-ground different from that of the EKG machine, or with an "antenna" such as the bed frame from which he is imperfectly insulated, 60-cycle artifact will appear in the tracing and will be proportional to the difference in potential-to-ground between the two components concerned. In such instances, the interference can be eliminated either by breaking the offending contact or by putting the external equipment at the same potential as the patient and the EKG machine by "grounding it" to the EKG machine; all machines come with a ground wire for this purpose. The problem of 60-cycle interference can almost always be controlled by following the instructions that come with the instrument, but sometimes a little detective work may be necessary to identify the problem. An unusual source, for instance, is a break in the patient cable, a problem that can be localized by process of elimination and verified fluoroscopically.

There is very little electrical hazard in the ordinary recording of electrocardiograms. If a patient who is connected to an EKG machine is connected at the same time to another device that derives power from house current and has a potential-to-ground substantially different from that of the EKG machine, current will flow through his body, but the density of the electrical field in the area of the heart will usually be so small that it will be insignificant. If there is a low-resistance pathway into the patient's heart, e.g., a saline-filled catheter in continuity with electrical equipment, the current density in the myocardium may be great enough to induce ventricular fibrillation. The use of monitors, electric beds, and other electric systems has increased this kind of risk to the patient as well as the operator.[380,396] When recording a tracing from a patient who is connected to other equipment, the other equipment should be disconnected from the power supply (unplugged — not just turned off) before the patient is connected to the EKG machine.

Calibration

Pressing the calibration (or standardization) button delivers exactly one millivolt to the recorder, and the deflection this produces serves as a reference point not only for amplitude but also for the response characteristics of the system. The instrument is adjusted so that this signal produces a deflection of 10 mm, and voltages are always expressed in terms of this scale; i.e., 10 mm = 1.0 mv. Because QRS complexes are often so large that they run off the chart, a switch is provided to cut the scale in half without adjusting the continuous amplitude control. It is important to recognize that it makes little difference at what amplification (gain) the tracing is recorded but that it must be known to the interpreter. This can be assured by calibrating each lead.

The shape of the calibration deflection is an indication of the response characteristics of the instrument (Figure 14-1). When properly adjusted, the pulse has sharp, square corners. If the stylus is overdamped — pressing too hard on the paper — the corners of the deflection will be rounded because higher frequencies cannot be recorded; if underdamped — too little pressure — spiked. Clinically important errors of interpretation may result from either over-damping or underdamping.[381-383] It is the reponsibility of the technician to recognize inappropriate response and to correct it by following the instructions that came with his machine, but if he does not, the interpreter must recognize it. With the introduction of each new model, stylus technology is improved, and the problem of over-damping and poor adjustment of the stylus/paper relationship lessens (see page 142).

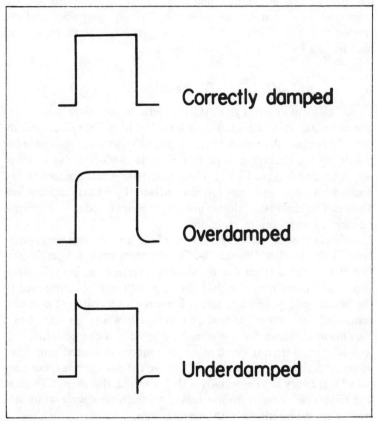

Figure 14-1. Damping. Calibration of the tracing with a square wave of one millivolt identifies not only the amplitude of a deflection but also the response time of the instrument.

Labeling the Tracing

A mislabeled tracing is worse in some ways than no tracing at all. Leads must be labeled clearly. Three-channel, automatic switching equipment takes care of this, as well as calibration, automatically. Single-channel machines not so equipped provide a marking stylus with which each lead can be coded individually during recording. Any code will do as long as it is understood by everyone concerned and labels the leads in a mutually exclusive fashion. A good one is dots for leads 1, 2, and 3, dashes for R, L, and F, and a dash followed by dots for precordial leads. The patient's name and identification number, as well as the date and time, should be recorded on each tracing at the time it is made when there is only one patient and one tracing at risk. It is also well for the technician to sign his tracings so that he can be identified if questions arise.

RECOGNITION OF TECHNICAL ERROR

Of all artifacts *60-cycle* AC interference is probably the most common, and its causes and their remedies have been discussed under "Grounding the Equipment" on page 137. It is recognized in the tracing by the occurence of perfectly regular deflections at a rate of 60 per second (Figure 14-2B). These may be of any amplitude in any lead and may or may not interfere materially with interpretation. They can be eliminated almost always, or at least reduced to insignificance, by appropriate grounding.

Muscle tremor is recognized by rapid, coarse, irregular variations in the baseline (Figure 14-2C). Beginners most frequently confuse it with the artifact due to 60-cycle interference, but it is much slower and more irregular than this, e.g. a "noise" as compared to the "hum" of 60-cycle artifact. It is simply a recording of potential generated in active striated muscle somewhere in the body. Parkinson's disease, for instance, may result in a characteristic pattern of muscle tremor much more pronounced in frontal leads than in precordial ones. The remedy is to have the patient relax, but people who are very sick, especially if they are cold, disoriented, in pain, and frightened, cannot always relax. A moderate degree of muscle tremor rarely interferes with interpretation.

Wandering of the baseline up and down is the result of motion of an electrode with relation to the skin and is more common in precordial leads than frontal ones because of the unavoidable motion of the chest with respiration (Figure 14-2D). The remedy is to be sure that the electrodes are attached securely but not so tightly as to cause dis-

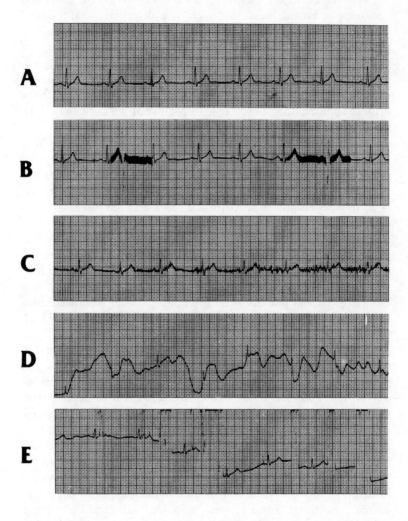

Figure 14-2. Common artifacts. A, normal tracing; B, intermittent 60-cycle interference; C, muscle tremor; D, wandering baseline due to instability of skin-electrode contact; and E, very abrupt deflections, instability of metal-to-metal contact.

comfort, and then to be sure that the patient is still. A moderate degree of wandering of the baseline is acceptable, especially if the patient is a small child, very ill, and uncooperative.

Very *abrupt deflections*, often all the way across the chart and occurring in bursts, mean that there is a defective metal-to-metal contact in the system (Figure 14-2E). The most common place to find this is in the connection of a lead wire to an electrode, and tightening of the binding screw will correct it. The only other place that it occurs with any frequency is within the patient cable itself; problems here may be localized by recognizing the leads in which the artifact appears, and fluoroscopic inspection of the cable may show the break directly.

Before direct-writing EKG equipment was available, time lines were projected on the film during recording, but the nature of modern equipment requires that they be inscribed before the paper is put into the machine. This means that the paper must move at exactly 25 mm per second in order for the space between two small lines on the graph to represent 0.04 sec. When tracings are recorded at *50 mm per sec*, and this is not recognized, they may be interpreted as showing marked bradycardia and prolongation of PR, QRS, and QT intervals and sometimes as suggesting drug or electrolyte effect. Inappropriate paper speed may be suspected easily enough if one knows the patient and his heart rate, but it cannot be proved from the tracing itself unless it includes 60-cycle artifact, which will look like 30-cycle artifact.

Indistinctness of the baseline, blurred, too light, or of varying width, is usually a result of improper relation between stylus and paper. The most common means of recording electrocardiograms today is with a heated stylus writing on heat-sensitive paper drawn tightly over a knife-edge so that only one point on the paper is in contact with the stylus at a given time (Figure 14-3). The method requires that the traverse of the stylus be exactly parallel to the surface of the writing edge and that proper pressure be applied across the whole chart. A dirty or bent stylus or one that is too hot can produce fuzziness of the trace, and an error in insertion of the paper can do the same thing. Some systems write with ink forced through a pointed stylus onto specially coated paper; others, a jet of ink so that the stylus does not touch the paper at all, and electrical-spark writers and carbon transfer techniques have been used.

Rectilinear conversion, correction for the fact that the stylus is actually describing an arc of a circle, is accomplished most frequently by the knife-edge method; other methods utilize a platen curved in the arc of the circle of which the stylus is a radius or use a system of levers to permit writing on a flat surface.

It has been noted that it makes no difference where electrodes are placed on arms and legs, but this is far from the case with precordial leads whose *electrodes must be placed accurately*. The positions for these have been described (see page 27), and it should be mentioned again that they are based on bony landmarks of the thoracic cage and do not vary with changes in soft tissues or with changes in body size and shape. Leads made from the right side of the chest in positions corresponding to those on the left are identified by the suffix R, e.g., V_3R, V_4R. V_1 and V_2 do not change names.

Perhaps the most common serious errors fall into the category of *"crossed leads"* and are made occasionally by even the best of

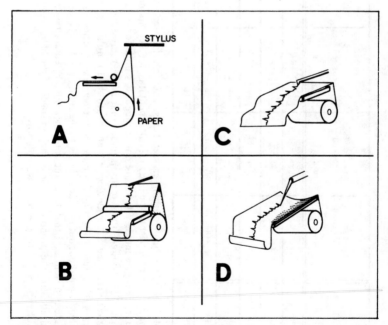

Figure 14-3. Types of stylus. Several combinations of methods of writing and of rectilinear conversion are in use in addition to those indicated here. The hot stylus in contact with heat-sensitive paper drawn tightly over a sharp edge as in A and B is the most common.

Lead	Correct connections	Arm leads crossed R↔L	Left leads crossed L↔F	Right leads crossed R→F	Arm and leg leads crossed ipsilaterally R→F L↔F	
I	+L -R	+R -L	+F -R	+L -F	+F -F	
II	+F -R	+F -L	+L -R	+F -F	+L -F	
III	+F -L	+F -R	+L -F	+F -L	+L -F	
aVR	+R -(L+F)	+L -(R+F)	+R -(F+L)	+F -(L+F)	+F -(F+L)	
aVL	+L -(R+F)	+R -(L+F)	+F -(R+L)	+L -(R+F)	+F -(F+L)	
aVF	+F -(R+L)	+F -(L+R)	+L -(R+F)	+F -(F+L)	+L -(F+F)	

Figure 14-4. Schema for identifying crossed leads. The right leg electrode is for grounding only and is equally effective no matter to which part of the body it is attached; it is not a component of any lead. As long as all three corners of the triangle are represented, V leads are not changed. R stands for the right arm, L for the left arm, and F for the inferior angle of the triangle (the symphysis pubis) that can be represented equally well by attachment of the electrode to either leg. The right leg electrode does not enter into the formula, e.g., when right arm leads are crossed, the R electrode comes to represent F (in addition to the F electrode attached to the left leg). Grounding is still by way of the right leg lead even though it is attached now to the right arm. In this setting, information from the right arm corner of the triangle is absent and that from the inferior angle, F, enters twice. When incorrect attachment of electrodes is suspected, identify the proposed error in the top space of the blank column and test the hypothesis by substituting in the formulae provided by the first two columns.

technicians. One way to catch them is by pattern recognition, but an easier and more useful way is to keep in mind that the possibility of error exists and to analyze tracings completely and logically.

Most beginners, given the hint that there is a technical error and asked to explain it, will say something like "The leads are crossed." Asked which leads, the answer will be "the limb leads," an incomplete explanation at best. Asked again, the response may be that lead I and lead II are crossed, a hypothesis that does not make sense at all in terms of recording but might explain an error of mounting and labeling. Part of the problem is that the word *lead* is used in electrocardiography in at least three senses; the concept of a dipole, the tracing itself, and the wire connecting the electrode to the machine. It is in this last sense that leads are crossed in recording.

If lead wires have been attached to the patient incorrectly, the tracing can still be interpreted if appropriate corrections can be made. Corrections are possible as long as all three corners of Einthoven's triangle are represented but not when two of the three lead wires are attached to the legs and thus represent a single point. There follows a list of the usual patterns of error in this field, each introduced by a description of the problem the electrocardiographer will recognize. Once suspected, substitution in a form such as that in Figure 14-4 may be used to test an explanation for crossed leads.

1) *Complexes in lead I are "upside down."* The arm leads are crossed; the left arm lead is on the right arm and vice versa. When this happens the polarity of lead I is reversed and the lead labeled II is really III, III is really II, and aVR and aVL are swapped. Lead aVF and the V leads are not changed. All the information is present, it simply needs to be viewed differently; correction is easy.

If the QRS is perpendicular to lead I (+90° or −90°), recognition may depend on orientation of P, and if there is atrial fibrillation (i.e., no P) it may be impossible to identify crossed arm leads — but in these circumstances it makes little difference.

2) *Lead I is flat.* Arm leads are on the legs and leg leads are on the arms. Remember that there are only three corners in a triangle; the lead to the right leg is for grounding (G) and does not relate to the tracing otherwise. A ground can be provided from any position on the body, and the right leg just happens to be the one that is used. When arm and leg leads are swapped, lead I is flat (really flat, not just small complexes, almost completely flat) because both electrodes involved are attached to the same angle of the triangle, the

symphysis pubis, and there is no difference between a point. The leads labeled II and III are both III but upside down. Only two angles of the triangle are represented, and the tracing, though not useless, is incomplete.

3) *Lead II is flat.* Right arm and leg leads are crossed. The trace in lead II is flat because both its electrodes are attached to legs, to the same point on the volume conductor, and there is no difference in potential between them. The lead labeled I is III upside down, lead III is valid, and the tracing is incomplete. If all the forces are directed to −30° or +150° in a normal tracing, a very similar finding will result, but the trace in lead II will not be absolutely flat.

4) *Lead III is flat.* Left arm and right leg leads are crossed. This is an unusual problem. Lead I becomes lead II; lead II is unchanged; and lead III is missing. The tracing is incomplete.

5) *Lead aVR, aVL, or aVF is flat.* A lead wire in the patient cable is broken. Modern patient cables with six precordial lead wires are more complex than earlier models and it is possible to get a tracing in leads I, II, and III, while a flat line is recorded in aVR, aVL, or aVF as a result of a fracture of the lead. If suspected, this can be established by fluoroscopy of the wire itself or by proper testing with a voltmeter. Often this problem is transient and difficult to identify when the break is not gross.

6) *Suggests inferior infarct.* When a Q3 raises the question of an inferior infarct in a patient who is thought not to have had one or when it is part of a tracing in which the electrocardiographer suspects error, consider the possibility that the left arm and leg leads are crossed. If there is a previous tracing, comparison with the present one will show the changes described. If there is only one tracing, that it suggests an inferior infarct but "just does not look right" may alert the electrocardiographer, a negative P3 may help but proof is not possible. Suspicion of this problem is an indication for repeating the tracing with special attention to lead placement.

When the left arm and leg leads are crossed, lead II is really lead I, I is II, and III is upside down. This is a two-edged problem: it may either simulate an infarct where an infarct is not present or obscure one where one is present — and it is much less easily suspected than the errors described above. It will help to remember that the sign of the P and T in lead III, as well as that of QRS, will be reversed. Lead III is often a "transitional" lead, i.e., its complexes are small and biphasic, since most of the forces are perpendicular to it, and tiny changes in orientation of the QRS will make qualitative changes in sign.

7) *Other errors can be made.* When a tracing is made on a single-channel machine with a single precordial lead wire, the lead selector switch may be left on aVF while the precordial electrode is placed properly but not turned on, and the result is that V_{1-6} are all aVF. A precordial lead may be swapped with any extremity lead, chest leads may be recorded in reverse order, V_{6-1}, or from the right side of the chest, and, if the patient cable has six precordial wires, they may be mixed in almost any combination. When V_1 and V_3 are transposed, for instance, the pattern of an anterior infarct can be very convincing unless one suspects the real problem.

8) *Errors of mounting and labeling.* A properly recorded tracing may be labeled incorrectly (including designation of the patient himself) or mounted incorrectly (upside down or in the wrong position on a preprinted form, for instance). Other possibilities exist, and it is not nearly so easy to predict them as in the case of errors of recording; awareness of the problem is the most important safeguard. If the tracing is analyzed and described completely, it will often become apparent that the leads as labeled cannot be correct. An important defense against errors in this category is to require that each lead be labeled and patient identification written on the tracing before it is trimmed for mounting.

Other Techniques

Telemetry means measurement from a distance; display of tracings at the central station in an ordinary monitoring unit is an example of its everyday use. The idea is not new; Einthoven wrote about it in 1906.[686] Electrocardiograms have been transmitted from the moon by radio, and similar systems are used increasingly for monitoring patients who are not confined to bed or who are at distant points in the hospital.[399] Another common example of telemetry is the transmission of electrocardiograms by telephone (Dataphone, facsimile), making prompt consultation available to physicians and patients even in areas remote from medical centers.[385] Acoustic-coupled methods for this were introduced about 1963, automatic facsimile systems have been common since the early 1970s, and the computer combines telemetry with analysis.

Tape recordings of electrocardiograms, using a portable unit worn by the patient as he goes about his regular activities, permits documentation of disorders of mechanism and, less frequently, of ST displacement. The tape is played back at a very rapid rate, and the information is analyzed by a system that permits real time reproduction of tracings for demonstration of selected events. This method, known as Holter monitoring after its inventor,[386,610, 611,679,680,685] is useful especially in patients in whom AV block or paroxysmal rapid heart action is suspected and, less clearly, for documentation of evidence of coronary insufficiency.

Fetal electrocardiography is useful sometimes when there is a question of fetal death, or one of twinning,[390,391] and a similar technique has been adapted for observation of the fetus during delivery.[392,474]

Multichannel recording with automatic switching of the leads and automatic calibration, now commonplace, diminishes the incidence of human error in recording and identification of tracings, lessens the material cost per tracing, speeds processing considerably,[393] makes it easy to leave a copy of the tracing on the ward, or with the patient, while one is returned to the heart station for processing, and promises to be standard for the foreseeable future. The use of six precordial lead wires introduces possibilities for mislabeling of precordial leads not found when a single one is used.

Vectorcardiography has been discussed on pages 9 and 36.

Body surface mapping produces a picture of the projection on the body surface of electrical events taking place within the heart and has several research applications including quantitative estimation of myocardial injury.[398,684]

The use of lead III made during *deep inspiration* has been proposed from time to time to help in evaluation of Q3, and sometimes will bring out disorders of cardiac mechanism,[394,489,496,532] but adds little.

Intracardiac tracings are of help sometimes in diagnosis of congenital heart disease[397] and can be used for placement of pacemakers and catheters.[472,682]

His bundle electrocardiography, direct recording from selected portions of the intracardiac conduction system, has contributed much to understanding of disorders of impulse formation and conduction but is very rarely necessary for clinical decisions in individual patients.[678,683]

An *esophageal* lead is useful in rare instances for identification of P waves.

CHAPTER XV

Miscellany

STRESS TESTS

A study designed to evaluate the reserve of a system is called a provocative, tolerance, or stress test; examples include the hepato-jugular reflux, the glucose tolerance test, and the group we are concerned with here, procedures that test the capacity of the coronary arteries to deliver more blood in response to an increase in demand. A stress test differs from a simple measurement in that it has two variables, challenge and response; both must be defined clearly, one fixed and the other validated by correlation with some other measure of the reserve in question.

Clinical Orientation

Given a patient with chest pain thought to be due to impairment of coronary blood flow, i.e., angina pectoris, and recognizing that the disease most likely to produce this is atherosclerosis, two distinct and easily separable components of the diagnosis must be considered, topography and etiology. The suspected lesion and its location, narrowing of the lumina of large coronary arteries, can be identified readily by angiography. There is no means short of biopsy to prove that the narrowing is due to atherosclerosis, but for practical purposes atherosclerosis is the only thing that produces such lesions and the clinical diagnosis is acceptable, especially if there are "risk factors" known to be associated with atherogenesis and there is evidence of arterial insufficiency in another vascular bed. Demonstration of arterial obstruction, however, does not establish that the physiologic lesion — inadequacy of perfusion of the ventricular myocardium — is present; it is for this that the electrocardiogram is useful, and transient ST-segment displacement is the hallmark.

Challenge

An ideal stress test would involve a single function specifically, and in the case of coronary blood flow this is not possible. With the exception of controlled reduction of inspired oxygen,[314] application of ice water to an extremity,[313] and narrowing of coronary lumina by ergonovine,[602-603] all challenges have depended upon increasing the demand for blood. Tachycardia induced by artificial pacing of the heart[315,316] has the advantage of not requiring understanding or physical action by the patient, of being easily controlled, and of being almost specific for the system in question, but it is complex, unpleasant, and has never been popular. Other methods have included even quizzes,[505] but nearly all have been in the form of exercise (requiring the cooperation of the patient), and have limits other than those imposed by the coronary circulation, e.g., obesity, arthritis, debility, and lung disease. There are circumstances in which unquantified exercise such as doing a few knee bends, climbing a flight of stairs, or walking in the corridor can give useful information to a doctor who knows the patient and understands the method, but for results that are reproducible and can be standardized the stimulus must be fixed. Except for those that use a bicycle ergometer, all the tests that have gained wide acceptance depend upon walking, a physiologic activity requiring no training and applicable to substantially the whole population at risk.

Criteria for quantification of the amount and type of exercise vary. The first widely used set of standards was derived by Dr. Arthur M. Master, who began his work in the 1920s and was still actively engaged in it at the time of his death in 1973. His first studies were concerned with physiology; the electrocardiographic aspect of the test was added later. Recognizing that almost everyone who walks also climb stairs, he devised a platform consisting of two steps, each 15 cm in height, and, over a period of years, determined by trial and error a standard number of trips over the steps to be accomplished in a precisely specified time.

Later investigators concerned with physical fitness and measurement of the capacity of individuals to do work developed other methods of exercise. These generally are subdivided into clearly defined increments, or stages, of time and work and depend upon the treadmill which, with its adjustable rate and inclination, permits a degree of fine tuning not available with the two-step technique.

Because heart rate correlates well with myocardial oxygen utilization, it is an important criterion in the graded tests — either as an end point, or target, defining the level of stress at which the EKG response is to be evaluated, or as a measure of response to exercise quantified by other standards. When angiography and surgery for coronary disease became available, the graded tests proved helpful for evaluation of the patient with angina before and after surgical intervention; a subject can serve as his own control, with his post-operative response compared to his response to the same stimulus before surgery. The nearest to standards for graded exercise are those described by Dr. Bruce and his associates for maximal stress, i.e., symptom limited,[566] and by Drs. Sheffield et al. for submaximal, i.e., rate limited,[630] but numerous modifications of these and others are in use.

Response

In the 1920s[564] it was observed that flattened displacement of the ST segment accompanies the pain of coronary insufficiency, and abundant experience since then not only has confirmed this but also has shown that the same finding may be chronic in patients who, though they may have coronary atherosclerosis, do not have angina, i.e., ST displacement is a more sensitive indicator of impairment of blood flow than is pain. This is one of the firmest laboratory evidences of functional change in all of medicine and is uncontroversial as a marker for coronary insufficiency; its usefulness is limited only by quantitative factors. Insufficiency is not an all-or-nothing phenomenon but a continuum, and the point at which it becomes significant is arbitrary.[530] Any definition of criteria for a positive response must fix two components, ST displacement and contour. ST *displacement* is defined as departure of the J *point* from the baseline and, because it is observed customarily in leads with positive QRS complexes, it is usually recognized as depression. The ST *contour* typical of subendocardial injury is described as "flattened" or "downsloping"; sometimes it is called "ischemic," but this is an interpretation rather than a description.

In 1958 Dr. Lepeschkin proposed a device for statement of both displacement and contour in a single figure, the QX:QT ratio,[325] and this was accepted by Dr. Master.[318,322] A line is drawn connecting the beginning of two contiguous QRS complexes in as flat as possible portion of the tracing (Figure 15-1) and the point at which the ST segment crosses this line is labelled X. The QX time is compared to the duration of QT, and a QX:QT ratio of greater than 50% defines both flattening and depression. Other definitions of the critical abnormality of contour include specified levels of the trace below the baseline at 0.06 or 0.08 sec after J, and still others can be used.[631] The limitation of all these is the limitation of human ability to define points — and the human tendency to express estimates with a degree of precision beyond the limit of the method; use of the QX:QT does not eliminate this problem but reduces it to estimation of a single number. Recently it has been proposed that increase in QRS amplitude following exercise may be a useful measurement in this difficult area.[551]

Elevation of ST[327,328] may be an abnormal response, and so may transient Q waves, some arrhythmias, and changes limited to the T or U. All of these may influence the experienced doctor who is studying the patient, but flattened ST depression remains the chief criterion of a positive test.

The need in all of these studies for a control 12-lead tracing made at rest is clear. Not only will it lessen the likelihood of subjecting a patient with a recent infarct to inappropriate exercise, but also will prevent misinterpretation of preexisting abnormalities as evidence of a positive response. There is general agreement that the more marked the displacement and flattening the greater the discrepancy

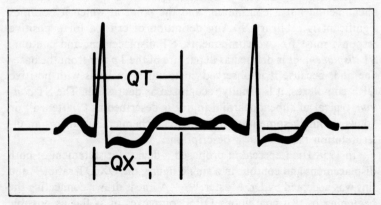

Figure 15-1. QX:QT ratio.

of coronary blood flow,[525,530,578] but specific values to define the point at which a response becomes positive remain controversial.

Validity

A laboratory study is useful only to the extent that it can be equated with disease, and in a stress test, once the challenge and the response by which it is to be measured have been agreed upon, the response must be related to some well-defined evidence of disease. Part of the reason for differences of opinion about exercise tests in patients with coronary disease is that the clinical side of the equation is defined differently in different studies. There must be clear differentiation between angina and coronary narrowing; the two are closely related but are not at all precisely the same.[558] About 40% of patients 40 years of age or older and free of clinical evidence of heart disease can be expected to have occlusion or severe narrowing of a major coronary artery,[567] and severe narrowing of coronary lumina occurs even in healthy young adults without symptoms.[559] In one study of American soldiers killed in action in their early 20s, 3% had occlusive lesions.[568] The difference between the disease process, atherosclerosis, almost ubiquitous in adult Americans and the basis for most angina, and the physiologic lesion itself, discrepancy of blood flow, must be identified. There may be angina without demonstrable coronary disease, and flattened ST displacement typical of coronary insufficiency is not rare in old people without clinical heart disease. Whatever criteria are used, false positives and false negatives occur, and the significance of a positive response in any test must be decided in the final analysis by the doctor responsible for the patient.

Procedures

The diagnosis of angina is made by history, and if the history is unequivocal no test is needed to support it. To subject an asymptomatic individual to a stress test for coronary blood supply may be justifiable when the interests of others are concerned and the candidate is willing to accept the risk of a false-positive response, e.g., application for life insurance or for a job as an airline pilot. The benefit to the applicant in such instances is obvious, but the risk of his becoming a patient as a result of the test should be recognized.

When the cause of chest pain is not clear but is suspected of being coronary insufficiency, the *Master test* can be helpful. Universally available, inexpensive, clearly defined, and almost devoid of risk, it may be ordered in the same sense that an electrocardiogram or chest film is ordered. It requires that a doctor examine a control tracing and approve the test, but the test itself may be conducted by a technician and reported by the electrocardiographer as positive or negative.

The only equipment needed is an EKG machine and a pair of steps, each nine inches high. A 12-lead tracing is made with the patient at rest and is inspected before he is allowed to exercise. The patient walks over the steps a specified number of times determined from a table (Figure 15-2) derived by Dr. Master from experience and based on age, weight, and sex.[319,320] Originally the exercise lasted 1.5 minutes, but the double test, twice the original number of trips and lasting 3 minutes, is now standard. A 15% increase in the number of trips was proposed in order to increase the precision of the results,[323] but this augmented test has not been used widely. If at any time during exercise the patient experiences chest pain, exercise is discontinued, and a tracing is made. Immediately upon completion of exercise leads 2 and V_{4-6} are recorded, and the same leads are repeated two and six minutes after exercise has been completed.

Much of the discussion about what determines positivity of a Master test is unnecessary; this was defined by Dr. Master, and a two-step test conducted by other standards is not a Master test, but the meaning of a positive or negative response remains a matter for interpretation. Changes in ST-T-U, the presence of ectopic beats, and/or disorders of AV conduction following exercise must be recognized, but the chief criterion by which response is defined as positive or negative is change in the ST segment as reflected in the QX:QT ratio. The prognostic significance of the response to any stress test is very limited, but a positive Master test is strong evidence in support of a clinical diagnosis of coronary insufficiency and a poor outlook, while a negative one correlates well with a good prognosis even when the subject has had an infarct.[563] In one study, 97% of patients with a negative double Master test were still well 30 months later, while 60% of those with a positive test had signs of ischemic heart disease and 10% were dead.[333]

A shortcoming of the Master test is that it does not take into account the physiologic reserve of the individual as a whole — his

TABLE 1

Trips Performed in Master Double (Three Minute) Two-Step Exercise Test*
Males and (Females)

Weight lb.	Age in Years												
	15-19	20-24	25-29	30-34	35-39	40-44	45-49	50-54	55-59	60-64	65-69	70-74	75-79
50-59	64(64)												
60-69	62(60)												
70-79	60(58)												
80-89	58(56)	58(56)	58(56)	56(54)	54(52)	54(48)	52(46)	50(44)	50(42)	48(42)	46(40)	46(38)	44(36)
90-99	56(52)	56(54)	56(52)	54(50)	54(48)	52(46)	50(44)	50(44)	48(42)	46(40)	44(38)	44(38)	42(36)
100-109	54(50)	56(52)	56(52)	54(50)	52(48)	50(46)	48(44)	48(42)	46(40)	44(38)	44(36)	42(36)	40(34)
110-119	52(46)	54(50)	54(50)	52(48)	50(46)	48(44)	48(40)	46(40)	44(38)	44(36)	42(36)	42(34)	40(32)
120-129	50(44)	52(48)	54(48)	52(46)	50(44)	48(42)	46(38)	44(38)	42(36)	42(36)	40(34)	40(32)	38(30)
130-139	48(40)	50(44)	52(46)	50(44)	48(42)	46(40)	46(38)	44(38)	42(36)	40(34)	40(32)	38(30)	36(30)
140-149	46(38)	48(44)	50(44)	48(42)	48(40)	46(38)	44(36)	42(36)	40(34)	40(32)	38(32)	36(30)	36(28)
150-159	44(34)	48(42)	50(40)	48(40)	46(38)	44(38)	42(36)	40(34)	40(32)	83(32)	36(30)	36(28)	34(26)
160-169	42(32)	46(40)	48(38)	46(38)	44(36)	44(36)	42(34)	40(32)	38(32)	36(30)	36(28)	34(26)	34(24)
170-179	40(28)	44(38)	46(36)	46(36)	44(34)	42(34)	40(32)	38(30)	36(30)	36(28)	34(28)	34(26)	32(24)
180-189	38(26)	42(36)	46(34)	44(34)	42(34)	40(32)	38(32)	36(28)	36(28)	34(28)	32(26)	32(24)	30(22)
190-199	36(24)	40(34)	44(32)	42(32)	42(32)	40(30)	38(30)	34(26)	34(26)	32(26)	30(24)	30(24)	28(22)
200-209		38(32)	42(30)	42(30)	40(30)	38(28)	36(28)	34(26)	32(24)	32(24)	30(22)	28(22)	28(20)
210-219		36(30)	42(28)	40(28)	38(28)	36(26)	34(26)	34(26)	32(24)	30(22)	28(22)	28(22)	26(20)
220-229		34(28)	40(26)	40(26)	38(26)	36(26)	34(24)	32(24)	30(22)	28(22)	26(20)	26(20)	24(18)

*Master, A. M. and Rosenfeld, I.: "The two-step exercise test brought up to date," New York J. Med., 61:1850, 1961.

Figure 15-2. Exercise for the Master test. A trip from the floor on one side of the steps to the floor on the other is considered a single trip; return to the starting point, a second trip.

physical fitness; to determine the amount of exercise on the basis of weight, age, and sex, is not so logical as to use a percentage of reserve[335] as the criterion. The best measure of the latter seems to be heart rate, and this is an important standard in *graded tests,* both maximal and submaximal[336,337,566] but not an important feature of the Master test.[338]

Graded tests often include continuous monitoring of several events, not just the electrocardiogram, *during* controlled, increasing degrees of exercise as well as later in the recovery period. A treadmill is still relatively large and expensive, and the risk to the patient of graded exercise testing, though very small, is probably greater than that of a Master test. Specific figures that would be comparable are hard to define. These tests can be used for the detection of coronary artery disease, for the initial diagnosis of angina, but observation of the patient during the procedure by a qualified cardiologist is a big factor in this setting. They have been validated mostly by correlation with angiographic evidence of coronary narrowing rather than with angina, and their most uncontroversial application is in evaluation of patients with angina before and after coronary artery surgery, and for determination of the level of work that can be undertaken by such patients safely. The bibliography includes references that will introduce one interested in the subject to its literature.[366,495,497,515,527,532,542,566]

Positive responses may occur in patients who do not have significant coronary narrowing and negative responses in those who do, no matter which test is used. Digitalis,[330,537] hyperventilation,[331,500] ventricular preexcitation,[332] right bundle branch block,[523,528,549,565] left bundle branch block,[499,523,528] electrolyte imbalance,[597] and mitral valve prolapse[502] may be the basis for a positive response and may interfere with interpretation. In one study 20%-30% of young women with no discernible heart disease had positive Master tests.[597] The doctor who is to translate the results of the test into patient care must understand its limitations and use it with the same constraint that he would any other laboratory procedure. Whether a positive response is to be called false or not depends, of course, upon the judgment of a physician. If positivity is to be correlated with subendocardial injury, proof is even more difficult than if it is to be correlated with angina pectoris, i.e., subendocardial injury *due to* coronary artery disease, much less with proof of the existence of coronary artery disease based on angiographic studies. False negativity is even more difficult to define, but beta blockers and treatment with nitrates may be factors here, as well as inadequacy of the exercise stimulus. When the cause of chest pain is in doubt, a positive stress test of any kind is strong evidence in support of the clinical diagnosis of coronary insufficiency and a negative one against it.

Summary

Stress tests designed to evaluate the reserve of the coronary circulation vary in quantitative standards and in the clinical events with which they have been correlated. All are helpful when interpreted by one who understands their limitations, but none is specific, and all are subject to false positives and false negatives. The primary doctor concerned with whether his patient with chest pain has angina will get useful information from a Master test; the cardiologist who must decide if a patient with angina is a candidate for surgery, evaluate the patient's response postoperatively, or advise him about the amount and type of exercise he should undertake will need a graded test.

THE DIGITAL COMPUTER IN ELECTROCARDIOGRAPHY

By the 1950s, it was apparent that the digital computer, capable of manipulating alpha-numeric data in tremendous volume, at great speed, and with near-perfect accuracy, was well suited for analysis of electrocardiograms. The linear, or analogue, information in a tracing is readily convertible to numbers that can be related quantitatively to clinical, autopsy, and experimental data that have been accumulated over the years and that are the very basis for the usefulness of electrocardiography. By the late 1960s computer analysis could be had anywhere by means of telephone connection to centrally located equipment and was soon in wide use, mostly in small community hospitals. It was not needed in hospitals with staff members who could interpret tracings, and in some of those where it had been instituted much of the original enthusiasm was lost when it was realized that, effective though the read-out was as an aid, the final interpretation still depended upon the doctor himself.[513,514,550,687] The EKG consultant began to be defined more clearly, and a second group of candidates for use of the computer was identified — those who must process many tracings in a day. It is this group that can use the method most effectively in the present state of its development — its rapid, consistent, and precise analysis eliminating not only the need for tedious measurement but also the human error inherent in it, leaving the doctor free to interpret.

Philosophy of programming and use of computers varies a bit, but to expect any program ever to eliminate professional judgment seems inappropriate. As experience accumulates, programs grow increasingly more effective, to be sure, but computer analysis is a screen, and the final decision as to what information is in a tracing will always depend upon the doctor.

There are two basic types of analysis programs, the "XYZ" or "orthogonal" and the 12-lead. The former is based on the hypothesis that all of the electrical information available from any system is inherent in that projected on three mutually perpendicular leads. This is true, of course, but the usefulness of this approach is limited by the ultimately empirical nature of electrocardiography and the fact that validation of data accumulated over the last 75 years all relates to Einthoven/Wilson methods. Programs based on analysis of 12-lead tracings have achieved the widest acceptance and probably will be standard for the foreseeable future.

There are differences among programs but they are small and similar to differences among competitive brands of automobiles; most of the limitations are common to all of them and are the limitations of human ability to digitize all features needed for interpretation, not those inherent in computers. These are especially clear in working with disorders of impulse formation and conduction. The tradition of including its meaning, as well as a description of its linear characteristics, in the definition of a curve, is difficult to get around, but the computer cannot be told to recognize a P wave as evidence of atrial activity—it must be told precisely what a P wave is in terms of its morphology and how to differentiate it from a bump or wiggle in the baseline. Similarly, to interpret a P wave preceding a QRS as "causing" that QRS is a matter of judgment. Even in tracings that show third-degree AV block, there are P waves before QRSs; the conclusion that there is or is not a causal relation between them is based on many factors. Contours, too, are often a matter of judgment; some patterns, left bundle branch block and classic myocardial infarction, for instance, can be described with considerable precision, but differentiation between whether an ST sags or does not sag is difficult to convert to a digital statement.

Evaluation of a deflection, a Q wave for instance, may depend upon awareness of the clinical problem and findings in previous tracings, again judgment. Comparison with serial tracings, not always just the most recent one, is an absolutely necessary part of interpretation, and no programs yet available can do this effectively. Work in this field is in progress but usefulness seems to be a long way in the future. Ordinary electrocardiograms, those recorded on paper but not on magnetic tape, cannot yet be analyzed by computer. This means that all computer analysis must be "on line," done in real time, planned in advance. Tracings may be recorded on tape at the time they are made and transmitted later to a computer, but those made already, or made on equipment not compatible with the computer, are not suitable for computer analysis.

The relative accuracy of programs is a matter that generates discussion. One view is that all are right all of the time; i.e., each responds in the way in which it has been instructed to respond. The question is whether the instruction, the programming, was correct. At this point we must recognize again the fact that clinical electrocardiography is an extremely empirical discipline. "Proof" of a disorder of AV conduction, for instance, would be almost impossible, and quantitative definitions of even such easily defined concepts as hypertrophy and infarction are arbitrary to say the least. The validity of a program is determined customarily by vote of a panel of experts — and some of them may be wrong.

AXIS DEVIATION

The expression "axis deviation" has presented a problem in electrocardiography since the beginning. By long-established usage "axis" refers to the frontal projection of the mean QRS expressed as an arrow, or vector, and "deviation" implies that this is beyond the range of normal — left when more counterclockwise than it should be, and right when more clockwise. The problem is the common treatment of axis deviation as if it meant heart disease even though there is lack of agreement as to how it should be measured and what the range of normal is.[53] The term is often used without statement of either of these but with the tacit assumption that everyone must understand it.

Left axis deviation (LAD), defined as a mean frontal QRS counterclockwise to −30° (see page 34), is a statistical abnormality that is often associated with heart disease[159,357-361] — but not always. This finding, when abnormal, may be due to one or more of several mechanisms. One explanation is impairment of conduction through the anterosuperior ramifications of the left bundle branch (left anterior hemiblock), but it may also reflect loss of muscle inferiorly (as with infarction), change in electrical characteristics of the volume conductor (pulmonary emphysema), or, probably, disproportionate increase in the mass of muscle depolarizing leftward and upward (left ventricular hypertrophy). Structural anomalies of the chest may produce left axis deviation, so may artificial pacemakers or poisoning with quinidine or potassium, and sometimes it is found in the absence of any demonstrable disorder.[419]

Not nearly so much attention has been paid to definition of right axis deviation, probably because extremes of right axis deviation are less common than those of left and because right ventricular overload is less likely to be a clinical problem than left. Many normal subjects will have a mean frontal QRS directed downward (+90°), and +105° is a good criterion for the clockwise limit of normal. Causes of *right axis deviation* include right ventricular hypertrophy, left posterior hemiblock, and structural changes in the chest. Right bundle branch block need not be associated with either right or left axis deviation but may be associated with either,[171] and left bundle branch block may or may not be associated with left axis deviation.[660]

It is best to indicate the position of the mean frontal QRS and to avoid the term axis deviation entirely.

VOLTAGE

Voltage is what the electrocardiogram measures, the difference in potential between two points on the body. There is a positive relation between the amplitude of a deflection (voltage) and the amount of energy it represents, but the relation is far from linear; to assume, for instance, that high QRS voltage means an increase in the size of the generator, ventricular hypertrophy, and that low voltage means the opposite is an important mistake. Myocardial mass is probably the largest single factor in determining the amplitude of a deflection[606] but by no means the only one; many others can be identified. The distance from myocardium to electrode is important, and the electrical properties of intervening tissues may vary and influence the shape and size of the curve. Recording equipment and technique are important considerations, and the amplitude of a deflection in a single lead depends on the direction of the force with relation to that lead as much as on its magnitude.

The volume of the ventricles, the amount of blood in them, is an important component of the problem, some studies showing increase in voltage with increase in volume[468,581,582] and some the opposite.[583] Myocardial ischemia has been found to diminish voltage[594] and to increase it,[591] and even myocardial infarction may increase the amplitude of the R wave,[692] but different definitions and methods are involved in these reports, and more than one interpretation can be supported in each case. Pressure itself, the result of flow versus resistance, may be an important variable, voltage being greater with greater pressure,[584,585] but it may be that this should be interpreted as evidence of work instead of pressure. Hemorrhage will lower voltage,[604] but the size of the deflection may be restored by replacing the lost blood volume with saline. Pericardial effusion is commonly found to diminish voltage and this may be a result of diminution of the volume of blood in the ventricles, low arterial pressure, increase in venous pressure,[587,589] and/or an insulating effect of the pericardial fluid.[581,590]

Flow through the ventricles as in hyperthyroidism[470,593] or anemia must be considered, and habitus has been identified as playing a role[592] probably related to heart-electrode distance.[469] The effects of mastectomy should be recognized.[204] Though not very important, race, sex, and age must be included in this list,[465,467,588] and emotional stress has been said to increase voltage.[586,593]

Criteria by which voltage may be designated as high or low are available in a wide range of choices. Sokolow and Lyon's definition of high voltage[293] as SV_1 plus RV_5 (or RV_6, whichever is taller) greater than 3.5 mv is probably the most widely used one and is a convenient point of departure for recognizing left ventricular hypertrophy (see page 126), but this value cannot be estimated meaningfully any closer than 0.5 mv. Low voltage is harder to define and generally less important; a definition that serves well is that voltage is low if the total QRS (from the top of the tallest deflection to the bottom of the deepest one in lead 1, lead 2, or lead 3) is less than 0.5 mv. In all cases calibration is 1 mv = 10 mm.

DRUGS AND ELECTROLYTES

Digitalis

The effects of digitalis on the electrocardiogram are not predictable, but the changes it may induce are characteristic enough to be of potential value.[341,608,609] The preparation of the drug (digoxin, digitoxin, or leaf) and the route of its administration make no difference in its electrocardiographic manifestations; slowing of AV conduction, enhancement of ectopic automaticity, shortening of QT, and modification of the ST-T contour.

Distinction should be made between evidence of digitalis effect and that of excess or toxicity.[480] An early change is shortening of the QT interval, a particularly useful finding because almost nothing else (but hypercalcemia) does this. Precise definition of short is not easy; a value less than 0.32 sec, at usual rates, is a signal that the possibility should be considered. The change in shape of ST-T cannot be predicted on any very rational basis, but a characteristic, symmetric sagging of ST in association with lowering of T voltage in leads with positive QRS complexes (Figure 15-2) is typical.

Any degree of AV conduction delay can be produced by digitalis but complete block is rare. Second-degree block is usually of the Wenckebach variety and should be thought of as evidence of toxicity, but first-degree AV block may be of little clinical significance.

Ectopic beats, either atrial or ventricular, may result from overdose, but these are common in the absence of digitalis and may even be controlled by it if they are the result of congestive failure, and nothing in the form of the beats will distinguish among these possibilities. Almost any ectopic mechanism, including frequent multifocal premature ventricular contractions, and even atrial fibrillation itself can be produced by digitalis,[342,343] but only two are common, and each represents a combination of impairment of AV conduction and enhancement of automaticity — "PAT with block" and acceleration of a junctional pacemaker.

"PAT with block" implies atrial tachycardia with second-degree AV block,[80,81] and distinction between it and ordinary atrial flutter is a bit arbitrary, mostly a matter of atrial rate and knowing that the patient has been taking digitalis. In "PAT with block" the atrial rate is typically about 200 while in flutter it is close to 300. The same pattern may result from slowing of a rapid atrial pacemaker by antiarrhythmic drugs, and it may be idiopathic.[82]

In a patient with atrial fibrillation, digitalis may block conduction at the superior end of the AV node (entrance block) with the result that an AV junctional pacemaker escapes and drives the ventricles at a regular rhythm at a rate of about 50 with no change in the QRS; with advancing degrees of digitalis toxicity the rate may be greater.[106] Atherosclerosis, recent myocardial infarction, various inflammatory diseases, and cardiac surgery may cause the same thing.

Quinidine and Other Drugs

The effects of *quinidine* on the heart are complex, and some of its actions are counter to others. Typically, though, the net result is slowing of both AV and IV conduction and diminution of automaticity — it slows everything. The electrocardiogram may show any degree of AV block, and there may be prolongation of the QRS, which may be mistaken for bundle branch block, hyperkalemia, or even for recording the tracing at 50 mm per second.[203,204,576] Theoretically, the vagolytic effect of quinidine may speed AV conduction while the direct effect slows atrial rate with the result that one-to-one conduction may occur in patients being treated for atrial flutter, so-called 1:1 flutter (see page 63), but this must be very, very rare.

Procainamide (Pronestyl) and *disopyramide* (Norpace) produce substantially the same effects as quinidine[203,598-601] and those of hyperkalemia (see below) are similar. *Propranolol* (Inderal) and *lidocaine* (Xylocaine) produce little change.[344,345] *Phenytoin* (Dilantin) may or may not have an effect on AV conduction; the subject is controversial.[203,346] Other drugs whose electrocardiographic manifestations may be important include *chloroquine* and *emetine*,[347] and some of the tranquilizers such as *thioridazine*.[348] *Doxorubicin* (Adrianmycin), an antineoplastic drug, produces cardiomyopathy in some subjects and this may be suspected from significant reduction of the QRS voltage in serial tracings,[631,632] a method used also to test for evidence of rejection in cardiac transplants.

Electrolytes

Two electrolytes, calcium and potassium, may cause characteristic changes in the electrocardiogram. *Hyperkalemia*[349] produces a pattern that when fully developed includes tall, symmetrical, peaked T waves with diffuse widening of the QRS (one of the few instances of change in the QRS as a result of a lesion other than an anatomic one), prolongation of PR, and, in the later stages, loss of identifiable P waves and reduction of the QRS-T to a smooth, continuous sine wave. There is a rough correlation between the intensity of the changes in the tracing and the concentration of potassium in the serum.[350] Hyperkalemia also may simulate left anterior hemiblock.[433]

Hypokalemia[349,351] causes lowering of T voltage, some depression of ST (in leads with positive QRS complexes), rounding of T, and merging of T with a prominent U. It may be difficult to differentiate U from T, but a dimple in the contour, usually seen best in right precordial leads, helps. Generally, if the QT interval is much greater than about 0.44 sec the possibility that a U wave is being included should be considered.

These patterns were useful before determination of the serum potassium level was routinely available, and they still may be helpful as guides to changes in the serum potassium level with treatment, e.g., a patient being treated for diabetic acidosis, but it is not often that the electrocardiogram will give the first clue to potassium imbalance.

The pattern of *hypocalcemia*[352] is seen often in combination with that of hyperkalemia. It is characterized by lengthing of the Q interval with flattening of ST; changes in the sign and contour of T are inconstant. With *hypercalcemia* up to about 16 mg/dl the QT is shortened, but above this it may be prolonged.[353] There is little change in the T wave. *Sodium* and *magnesium* and other electrolytes produce little change in the electrocardiogram,[349] and changes in *pH* alone produce no recognizable change.[354]

It should be remembered always that a T wave may vary in only three ways — amplitude, sign, and duration — and that almost anything can influence at least one of these. Overinterpretation of EKG findings as evidence of electrolyte imbalance is not likely to produce harm, since the diagnosis can be verified, a situation very different from suggestion of anatomic diagnoses such as left ventricular hypertrophy or myocardial infarction, which cannot be "ruled out" by any means presently available.

PULMONARY DISEASE

Disease of the lungs may produce abnormalities in the electrocardiogram by way of changes in the intrathoracic volume and/or electrical properties as with pulmonary emphysema,[639,642] increase in resistance to outflow from the right ventricle, impairment of oxygen supply, and other less easily identifiable means such as pain. These occur in various patterns and may influence mechanism, structure, or function, either selectively or in combination.[640,641]

Disorders of mechanism are usually of atrial origin and factors other than the lung disease may be contributory, e.g., coronary atherosclerosis, pericardial metastases.[438] If there is increased resistance to right ventricular outflow, evidence of right ventricular enlargement (dilatation, hypertrophy, see page 126) is easy to understand, and so is the "unmasking" of an intraventricular conduction defect. Overload of the right ventricle is sometimes responsible for evidence of right atrial enlargement even when the ventricular lesion itself is not recognizable in the tracing. This can be attributed to an increased load on the atrium as a result of loss of compliance by the overworked right ventricle. The S1, 2, 3 pattern (see page 133) may be normal or give evidence of right ventricular enlargement of atypical right bundle branch block; interpretation is often arbitrary and dependent upon factors other than the tracing itself. Right atrial enlargement in these circumstances is evidence in favor of right ventricular enlargement, and PAC may have a similar meaning.

Nonspecific ST-T abnormalities are just that, nonspecific. They may be the only manifestation of any of the forms of lung disease. Prominence of Q waves in leads 2, 3, and F is particularly common in patients with lung disease, a pattern that may be indistinguishable from that of an old inferior infarct. There is no really satisfactory explanation for this, and it may present a difficult problem when the complaint is chest pain. A picture suggesting an old anterior infarct may be produced, too, probably by dilatation of the right ventricle.[614] The frontal QRS axis may be oriented in any direction including leftward and upward as with left anterior hemiblock,[437] presumably as a result of change in intrathoracic conductance as a result of replacement of tissue by air. A classic pattern characterized by a smooth curve from the peak of an accentuated P wave in leads 2, 3, and F to that of a low and rounded T results from a combination of right atrial enlargement of ST-T abnormalities and has been attributed to pulmonary emphysema.[639] Pulmonary embolism may produce any of the patterns described above, but findings due to it will always be transient, lasting no more than hours or days.

ELECTRICAL ALTERNANS

Electrical alternans is an unusual finding in which the amplitude of a deflection, sometimes even its sign, changes every other beat, i.e., alternates. It is seen most frequently in the QRS but may involve any component of the tracing selectively or in combination with others. There is a temptation to attach hemodynamic significance to alternation similar to that of pulsus alternans, and it is seen sometimes with pericardial effusion, but the mechanisms responsible for it are not at all clear and neither is its meaning. In the case of pericardial effusion, when alternation usually involves all components of the tracing, it may be related in some way to a pendulum-like motion of the heart within the fluid, but the more important abnormality probably occurs at the cellular level. Electrical alternans is not a very important finding in the present state of our knowledge.[471,545,634-638]

NERVOUS SYSTEM

There may be a cause-and-effect relationship between events in the nervous system and changes in the electrocardiogram.[362-365,503,595] EKG abnormalities resulting from CNS lesions, especially tall and peaked T waves, are mostly in the ST-T complex. These may be either positive or negative in precordial leads and must be differentialted from those of hyperkalemia and coronary insufficiency, but peaking of T is also common in normals. Seizures suggesting intracranial disease may be due to third-degree AV block (Stokes-Adams attacks), and the muscular dystrophies may involve the heart and simulate myocardial infarction very closely (see page 121).

BLUNT TRAUMA

Blunt trauma to the chest (e.g., automobile accidents, football injuries) may produce any EKG abnormality from nonspecific ST-T changes through disturbances in mechanism to atrioventricular and intraventricular conduction defects and even myocardial infarction depending upon the location and extent of the lesion. Most of these will be transient since they are presumably related to edema, extravasation of blood, or other intracardiac results of contusion that resolve in time.[205,252,271,366-369]

CONGENITAL HEART DISEASE

In congenital heart disease the electrocardiogram may yield helpful information in one or both of two ways; it may point to one or more chambers as overloaded or it may fit into a pattern, logical or not, that experience has shown to be associated with specific lesions.[372-374] Texts of cardiology are good sources of information on this subject, and the electrocardiographic patterns are usually discussed under the headings of the individual lesions.

PROLONGED QT SYNDROMES

It is during restoration of the polarized state in the ventricular myocardium and its conduction system that the T and U waves are written. The time required for this process would logically be measured from the beginning of the QRS to the end of the U, but U waves are small and their termination ill-defined and the QT interval, the time from the beginning of the QRS to the end of the T, is used instead. Almost the only thing that speeds repolarization and that has clinical significance is digitalis, but it can be lengthened by many, many things and because of the slope of the end of the T wave the range of normal cannot be called very close. Prolongation of QT is a common, and usually nonspecific, abnormality.

In 1957 Jervell and Lange-Nielsen described a constellation of findings including a long QT interval, syncopal attacks, and congenital deafness in four siblings three of whom died suddenly.[695] Later Romano et al. and Ward noted similar findings in the absence of deafness, and other patients have been described who had QT prolongation and life-threatening arrhythmias but without evidence of a hereditary basis for it. The serious problem common to all is syncope due to paroxysmal ventricular fibrillation or electrical instability, and the hypothesis is that the prolonged QT, or QT-U, somehow reflects the basic lesion, which is probably neurohumoral or enzymatic. Several reviews of the syndromes have been published.[509,657,689,690]

CHAPTER XVI

Description and Interpretation of the Tracing

This chapter is a summary of all that has gone before. It is arranged in the form of a guide, an algorithm, for the analysis, description, and interpretation of a tracing. The beginner who wants to learn by doing can use it to introduce himself to the subject, and the experienced electrocardiographer may find in it a stimulus to re-examine his own approach. What one brings to the study will make a difference in what he gets out of it and how he uses it, but the information in the tracing itself is the same whether the student is a technician or a cardiologist; most of it can be extracted by either, but only a doctor can interpret it.

There are two ways to handle an electrocardiogram. The patient's doctor, having taken the history, examined him, and reviewed the x-ray and other laboratory studies, may look at it, recognize that it supports his clinical evaluation (or at least does not contradict it), and proceed with treatment without recording anything at all or noting only that the findings are "compatible with" his diagnosis; this approach is practiced widely but has obvious limitations. A better method calls for orderly analysis, identifying and describing each of many components, noting change since previous tracings, and stating an interpretation, all in such a manner that another electrocardiographer can tell from the description how the conclusion was reached and why other possible explanations were rejected. This method provides a firm base for the beginner and is necessary for the doctor who interprets tracings for others. It requires clear differentiation between what one sees in a tracing and what one thinks it means, an important distinction and one easily overlooked.

There are three areas in which abnormality may be found:

mechanism ("rhythm"), structure (depolarization), and function (repolarization) — perhaps a fourth, patterns. Electrocardiographic identification of the *mechanism* of the heartbeat is one of the most exact of all clinical methods, amounting almost to definition, the QRS contains information about the *structure* of the ventricular myocardium and/or its conduction system (the P wave has a similar relation to the atria but presents less detail for analysis) and the ST-T-U reflects *function,* metabolism, physiology. Specificity diminishes and sensitivity increases from the QRS through ST to T and U.

Just as one follows a routine for physical examination, relates the findings to the history, laboratory, and previous findings, and makes a diagnosis with three components — topography, etiology, and manifestations — so with the electrocardiogram. He determines rates, intervals, orientation, displacement, and contour, relates the findings to the history and to previous tracings and other laboratory data, and makes an interpretation with three components — mechanism, structure, and function. The worksheet (Figure 16-1) has been designed to help in this process. The order in which information is extracted is not important but the order in which it is presented is, just as when one writes up the findings at physical examination. Beginners should work with real tracings and submit their descriptions and interpretations to an experienced electrocardiographer for comment.

Begin by looking at the whole tracing as you might look at a photograph of a familiar face; take it all in at a glance without conscious analysis of detail. This is done most easily if all 12 leads are mounted in a standard format on the same side of the same page. Starting with the big picture helps prevent becoming lost in minutiae, but analysis must follow, digitization and description of the several features, and, finally, synthesis of a diagnosis. Before one is through he must avail himself of whatever information he thinks he needs to make his interpretation most useful to the patient, and change his mind as many times as necessary if new information is presented.

Basic Measurements

1) *Ventricles* (QRS, see page 45)

Measure the ventricular *rate.* This can be done conveniently by using a meter based on three cycle-lengths or by counting the beats in six seconds and multiplying by ten (the lines in the margin of the paper are three seconds apart). When the rate is very rapid it may be necessary to estimate it by dividing one cycle length into 60 seconds (Figure 16-2). Consider the QRS *rhythm*. Is it regular? Irregular? Consistent? Inconsistent? Identify the *locus* from which ventricular depolarization proceeds. Is it supraventricular (narrow QRS complexes except when there is an intraventricular conduction defect)? Ventricular (wide QRS complexes)?

2) *Atria* (P waves, see page 44)

Determine the atrial *rate* by counting P waves. If the baseline is flat or fibrillary (not the same between any two consecutive pairs of QRS complexes in a given lead), the rate cannot be counted and this should be noted. What is the *rhythm* of the atrial complexes? Identify the *locus* of the pacemaker for the atria. Are the P waves of normal contour and orientation? Are they inscribed retrograde? Do they precede the QRS complex? Follow it? If no atrial activity is identifiable, note this.

3) *PR interval* (see page 45)

The PR interval is estimated in the lead in which it is longest *and* can be seen clearly, measuring from the beginning of the P to the beginning of the QRS (whether the first wave in that complex is a Q or an R). In adults with heart rates between 50 and 100, it does not exceed about 0.20 sec normally, but it cannot be called any closer than about 0.02 sec, and durations greater than 0.20 sec are not unusual in healthy people without heart disease (see page 77). If the PR varies, no figure should be entered here.

4) *QRS duration*

Measure the width of the QRS in the lead in which it is widest *and* in which its beginning and end can be identified most clearly, usually a right precordial one. In the normal adult the QRS duration is about 0.06 to 0.08 sec with 0.10 the upper limit of normal. It can be estimated usefully no closer than about 0.02 sec.

5) *QT duration*

The length of the QT is determined in the lead in which it is longest and can be defined satisfactorily. It is measured from the beginning of the QRS to the end of T and should be read to within about 0.04 sec. The usual value in adults with heart rates between 50 and 100 is 0.36 to 0.40 sec (Figure 16-3). A figure in excess of 0.44 suggests that a U wave is merged with the T, a common event and usual-

EKG WORKSHEET

Name:_____, Number:_____, Date tracing made:_____

I. Basic Measurements

Rate/min.: Atrial_____, Ventricular_____, PR 0._____sec., QRS 0._____sec., QT 0._____sec.

II. Mechanism
Atrial   AV   Ventricular
pacemaker:_____, conduction:_____, pacemaker:_____

III. Depolarization (structure)

P:_____

QRS: Mean frontal_____°, R:S V1_____:_____, R:S V6_____:_____, Contour_____

IV. Repolarization (function)

ST: | Displacement (J, a point)_____
    | Contour (a line)_____

T: Mean frontal_____°; Precordial,_____V1,_____V2,_____V3,_____V4,_____V5,_____V6

Amplitude and Contour_____

U: _____

V. Miscellaneous

QRS-T Angle: Frontal_____°; Horizontal_____°; Changes since previous tracing_____

VI. Interpretation

Mechanism:_____

Depolarization (structure):_____

Repolarization (function):_____

Other:_____

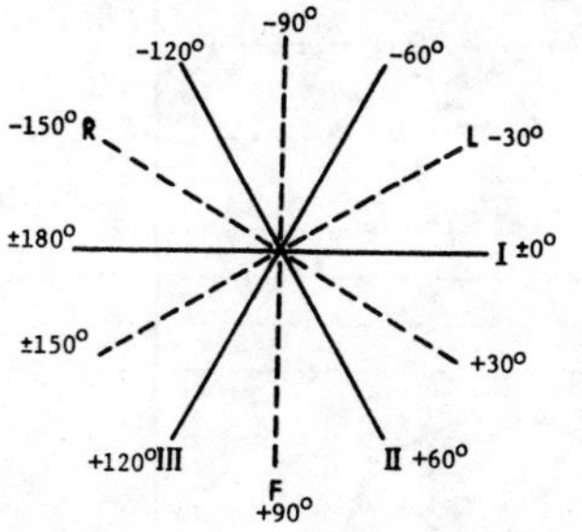

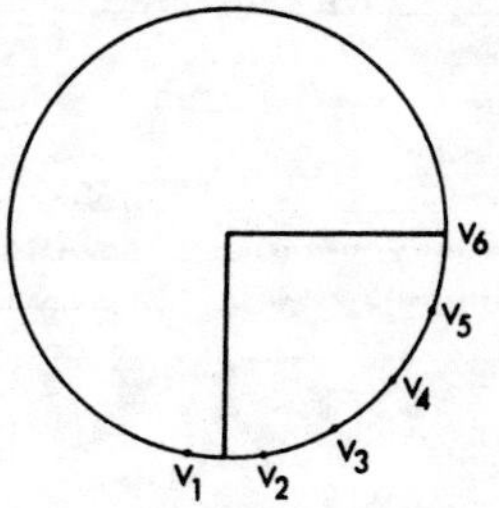

VII. Interpreted by:_____, Date:_____

Figure 16-1A. Work sheet for analysis of an electrocardiogram. Chapter 16 considers this form (or algorithm, or direction for problem solving) in some detail. It may be considered a summary of the whole book in application. Examples of its use are shown in Figure 16-1B.

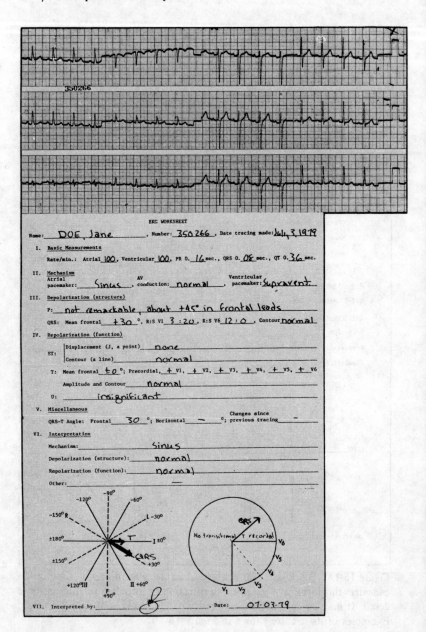

Figure 16-1B.

EKG WORKSHEET

Name: ROE Richard , Number: 288570 , Date tracing made: July 3, 1979

I. Basic Measurements

Rate/min.: Atrial — , Ventricular 130, PR 0. — sec., QRS 0. 08 sec., QT 0. — sec.

II. Mechanism

Atrial pacemaker: fibrillation, AV conduction: Variable, Ventricular pacemaker: Supra vent.

III. Depolarization (structure)

P: none

QRS: Mean frontal —75°, R:S V1 0 : 1 , R:S V6 2 : 8 , Contour normal

IV. Repolarization (function)

ST: Displacement (J, a point) none

Contour (a line) related to T—see below

T: Mean frontal +120°; Precordial, ± V1, neg V2, neg V3, ± V4, + V5, + V6

Amplitude and Contour low V5-6, contour not remarkable

U: not identifiable

V. Miscellaneous

QRS-T Angle: Frontal 165 °; Horizontal — °; previous tracing — changes since

VI. Interpretation

Mechanism: Atrial fibrillation

Depolarization (structure): Left anterior hemiblock

Repolarization (function): Not remarkable

Other: Precordial QRS progression is unusual

VII. Interpreted by: _____ , Date: 07-03-79

ly confirmed easily by identifying the U in a lead where its union with the T produces a "dimple."

Relationship Between Atria and Ventricles

While rate and rhythm of P and QRS can be determined with satisfactory objectivity, the locus of the pacemaker for each and the

1	2	1	2	1	2
77.5	77.5	56	107	34	176
77	78	55	109	33	182
76	79	54	111	32	187
75	80	53	113	31	193
74	81	52	115	30	200
73	82	51	117.5	29	207
72	83	50	120	28	214
71	84.5	49	122.5	27	222
70	86	48	125	26	230
69	87	47	127.5	25	240
68	88	46	130	24	250
67	89.5	45	133	23	261
66	91	44	136	22	273
65	92.5	43	139	21	286
64	94	42	143	20	300
63	95	41	146	19	316
62	97	40	150	18	333
61	98.5	39	154	17	353
60	100	38	158	16	375
59	101.5	37	162	15	400
58	103	36	166.5	14	428
57	105	35	171.5	13	461

Figure 16-2. Relation between cycle length and heart rate per minute. From Ashman and Hull, *Essentials of Electrocardiography,* 2nd. ed., 1941, courtesy of Dr. Edgar Hull. The rate is opposite the cycle length expressed in hundredths of a second.

causal relationship between them, if any, are necessarily matters of judgment (see page 55). Unless there is a clear statement to the contrary, ventricular complexes are assumed to derive from whatever focus has been identified as driving the atria. Analyze the relationship between Ps and QRSs. Is it predictable? Repetitive? Consistent? Regular? Irregular? Is there AV block (see page 50)? Ectopic impulse formation (see page 50)? The nomenclature of disorders of impulse formation and conduction often include illogically derived jargon that blurs distinction between observation and judgment, but it is possible to describe the events in plain English.

Depolarization

1) *P wave*

The most important feature of the atrial complex is that it be recognized. A P wave (see page 51) is a small deflection usually oriented downward and to the left with an initial component directed anteriorly and a terminal one posteriorly, i.e., usually positive in leads 1, 2, L, F, and V_6. A small notch is common and PV_1 is likely to be biphasic with the initial component positive and the terminal one negative. Right atrial enlargement produces tall, peaked P waves in leads facing the inferior aspect of the heart (2, 3, and aVF); left atrial enlargement, increased prominence of notching and, especially, of terminal negativity of PV_1 (see page 123). Retrograde depolarization of the atria reverses the polarity of the frontal P so that it is negative in leads 2, 3, and F (see page 123)

2) *QRS complex*

Orderly analysis of the ventricular complex is of special significance because it is here that diagnoses of structural abnormalities are made — diagnoses that usually cannot be proved or disproved but have important prognostic significance and affect the patient's well-being.

The *duration* of QRS and its *rate* and *rhythm* have been noted already. Its *orientation* in the frontal plane, the *axis* or the mean frontal QRS, is identified as a function of its net area and can be determined quickly and easily by inspection. The mean frontal QRS is perpendicular to the lead in which its net area is most nearly zero and parallel to the one in which this value is greatest. Its position can be estimated to within about ±15°, and the normal range is between approximately +90° and −30° (see page 34). If the complexes are biphasic in all leads (S1, S2, S3) or too small to justify meaningful analysis, note this and do not imply precision beyond the limit of the method by citing numbers. Einthoven's premises do not apply to the horizontal plane, and there is no standard reference figure for this projection; the direction of forces cannot be indicated by numbers as

| Cycle Lengths Sec. | Heart Rate per Min. | Men and Children Sec. | Women Sec. | Upper Limits of Normal | |
				Men and Children Sec.	Women Sec.
1.50	40	0.449	0.461	0.491	0.503
1.40	43	0.438	0.450	0.479	0.491
1.30	46	0.426	0.438	0.466	0.478
1.25	48	0.420	0.432	0.460	0.471
1.20	50	0.414	0.425	0.453	0.464
1.15	52	0.407	0.418	0.445	0.456
1.10	54.5	0.400	0.411	0.438	0.449
1.05	57	0.393	0.404	0.430	0.441
1.00	60	0.386	0.396	0.422	0.432
0.95	63	0.378	0.388	0.413	0.423
0.90	66.5	0.370	0.380	0.404	0.414
0.85	70.5	0.361	0.371	0.395	0.405
0.80	75	0.352	0.362	0.384	0.394
0.75	80	0.342	0.352	0.374	0.384
0.70	86	0.332	0.341	0.363	0.372
0.65	92.5	0.321	0.330	0.351	0.360
0.60	100	0.310	0.318	0.338	0.347
0.55	109	0.297	0.305	0.325	0.333
0.50	120	0.283	0.291	0.310	0.317
0.45	133	0.268	0.276	0.294	0.301
0.40	150	0.252	0.258	0.275	0.282
0.35	172	0.234	0.240	0.255	0.262

Figure 16-3. Normal QT intervals and the upper limit of normal. From Ashman and Hull, *Essentials of Electrocardiography*, 2nd. ed., 1941, courtesy of Dr. Edgar Hull.

it can in the standard 360° reference frame of the frontal plane. The precordial QRS is described instead by recording the height of the R and the depth of the S (adjusted to a standard of 1.0 mv = 10 mm) in V_1 and in V_6. The range of normal is very wide, but the complex is usually predominantly negative in V_1 and positive in V_6.

The relation between QRS and T has been estimated already in the frontal projection and must be evaluated in the horizontal plane, too, in order to have information in three dimensions. This can be done by assuming a value of 20° for the angle between contiguous precordial leads and identifying those to which the QRS and T are perpendicular (see above and page 39). This requires locating a transitional zone for *both* QRS *and* T, and when this cannot be done this approach will not work. The importance of estimating the relationship between QRS and T in the horizontal plane is to emphasize that we are dealing with three dimensions; the QRS-T angle may be small in the frontal projection, for instance, but large in the horizontal or vice versa.

Voltage, amplitude, is said to be low if the distance from the top of the R wave to the bottom of the S is not at least 0.5 mv in lead I, lead II, or lead III, an observation that rarely means much but must be noted (see page 160 for discussion of factors influencing voltage). The only reason for identifying the upper limit of normal is that high voltage may be a reflection of ventricular hypertrophy. The sum of SV_1 and RV_5 (or RV_6, whichever is taller) does not exceed 3.5 mv in most normals. This figure cannot be called any closer than 0.5 mv, though, and 4.0 is not necessarily an abnormal figure by itself out of clinical context. Left ventricular hypertrophy must be considered seriously at 4.5 and above 5.0 it becomes probable (see page 126). The recognition of right ventricular hypertrophy is more complex and less easily identified by a few numbers; basically, the more anteriorly the QRS forces are directed the more likely it is that there is right ventricular hypertrophy. In the full-blown picture the QRS complex in V_1 is predominantly positive while there is still a prominent SV_6 (see page 126).

The QRS *contour* in normals is clean and smooth and typically has a small initial deflection opposite a large terminal one, i.e., there is a small, clean Q wave in leads in which the QRS is mostly positive, and a small, clean, initial R in those in which it is negative. Abnormalities of contour may involve the initial part of the complex selectively, or the terminal part, or they may distort the whole thing. The most important cause of deformity of the first part is scarring of the myocardium, and this is usually a consequence of infarction — but not always (see page 120). Ventricular preexcitation can do the same thing (see page 82) and so can an increase in mass of muscle in the ventricular septum (see page 120); normal overlaps abnormal to a large extent. These early abnormalities usually take the form of a Q wave that is abnormal in either duration and/or contour or by virtue of its presence where a Q does not belong. Late QRS abnormality is typical of right bundle branch block (terminal forces are broad and slurred and directed to the right and, especially, anteriorly) (see page 85), and diffuse abnormality usually implies either left bundle branch block or more than one lesion (see page 87).

Repolarization

The atria must repolarize after each depolarization, and, at least theoretically, there must be a T_a (or P_t) wave, but this is not identifiable and is rarely, if ever, of clinical significance. For practical purposes, in EKG parlance the term repolarization implies repolarization of the ventricles, the T or ST-T complex (see page 101), and sometimes a U wave.

The nomenclature of ventricular repolarization is confusing. The whole process can be identified properly as T, but in practice it is usually subdivided into a proximal component of low frequency and amplitude, basically horizontal, the ST segment, and a distal one of greater frequency and amplitude that can be thought of as vertical, the T. This subdivision has come about because experience demonstrates that information of differing degrees of importance to the patient can be identified this way. It should be kept in mind that when one says ST segment it is clearly understood that he means the proximal part of the curve selectively, while T may mean *either* the distal part alone *or* the whole curve. This use of a single word to have more than one meaning is not unusual at all but is confusing unless recognized; when the whole curve is implied, uncertainty can be eliminated by speaking of the ST-T complex.

The characteristics of normal must be described before abnormality can be discussed. This is difficult to do for the ST-T in anything like a quantitative sense but can be approximated satisfactorily as follows. At the end of the QRS the trace is at or very close to the baseline (see page 48). As repolarization progresses it departs from that level at an increasingly rapid rate until a maximum deflection is reached, and there follows a relatively steep return to the baseline. A small, rounded wave may follow, the U, and this may be of either the same sign as the T or opposite. Note that whether the trace is above or below the baseline is not part of this description. Positivity or negativity is not an inherent characteristic of the repolarization process, but is an important part of describing it in a specific view (lead). In the normal heart the direction of repolarization is very close to that of depolarization (see page 19), left, down, and back, which is to say that in leads in which the QRS is completely positive the T will usually be positive also. With this description of normal as a point of departure, abnormalities can be discussed; judgment based on experience will often be the determining factor in deciding whether a given complex is normal.

Abnormalities of the *ST segment* can be divided into those of displacement and those of contour, and either or both may be present (Figure 16-4). *Displacement* is defined by the *level* of the *point* at which the ST can be distinguished from the QRS (the juncture of the QRS and ST, the "J point") as related to the level of the PQ segment (see page 44 for discussion of baseline). J may be above or below PQ, and the lead in which displacement is seen must be indicated as well as the sign of the displacement. Precisely how far from the baseline J must be to be called abnormal cannot be stated absolutely. It is commonly a bit elevated in right precordial leads in normal tracings, especially when the T is tall in those leads, and definition of the "point" itself entails judgment, since it is really a small area rather than a point. If ST contour is abnormal, displacement assumes more significance than when it is normal.[456] For practical purposes significant ST displacement can be equated with myocardial injury (see page 107).

The *contour* of the ST is the *shape* of a *line,* and abnormality can be described satisfactorily in most cases as sagging or arching or flattening. Think of the perimeter of a coin; its lower border can be seen as sagging, its upper as arching, and, viewed on edge, as flattened, but these all represent different aspects of the same curve. Contour is an intrinsic characteristic of the line written during ventricular repolarization: describing it can be compared to describing an object as spherical, a quality that does not require statement of the view from which the observation is made. This differs from description of displacement which, like indicating the movement of an object from one point to another, requires statement of direction and extent to be complete.

The *T wave,* the terminal component of the ST-T complex, is principally a vertical phenomenon and abnormality may be recognized in its amplitude, sign, or combinations of these plotted against time, i.e., contour.

The *duration* of repolarization has been measured as the QT interval, a value that includes the relatively small and fixed time of depolarization during which repolarization begins but cannot be seen, but is mostly a measure of the time required for repolarization, electrical systole. Almost any change makes it longer than normal but digitalis effect and hypercalcemia may shorten it.

Spatial *orientation* of the T is recognized in the same way as that of the QRS, by estimation of the mean area under the curve and its projection on the appropriate lead system (see page 34). Its frontal projection is expressed in degrees and its horizontal one by noting whether it is positive, isoelectric, or negative in each of the precordial leads. If T voltage is very low, this should be noted and no attempt made to assign number values.

Whether the *amplitude* of T, its voltage, is to be interpreted as great or small is determined by comparison to the amplitude of QRS, and whether it is normal or not is a matter of judgment that calls for experience. Generally, in leads in which the QRS is almost completely unidirectional the amplitude of the T will be at least 10% that of the QRS and of the same sign. Unusually high T voltage is more difficult to define; tall T waves may be abnormal (see page 107) but usually are not; low T voltage is often a nonspecific abnormality. T is commonly positive in right precordial leads with negative QRSs.

The *U wave* is a wide deflection of low amplitude following the T and usually of the same sign as the T. It can be identified in most tracings, especially in right precordial leads, but is not described routinely unless prominent.

Miscellaneous

1) *QRS-T angle*

The spatial relationship of forces generated during depolarization and those generated during repolarization, the QRS-T angle, is one of the most fundamental observations to be noted in analysis of the tracing. Its projection in the frontal plane normally does not exceed about 45° (but remember the limits of the method of determination of each of the components) and in the horizontal plane about 60° (see page 101).

2) *Comparison to previous tracings*

Whether findings are stable or unstable and, if changing, whether the nature of the change is toward normal or away from it can be recognized only by comparison with previous tracings, and this is a necessary part of the interpretation of every tracing when previous tracings are available. When findings are equivocal and the clinical problem is confusing, controls may be of much value; the potential for use as a control is one of the most important reasons to make most electrocardiograms.

3) *Artifacts*

Occasional technical errors are inevitable and this fact must be kept in mind. The most common serious ones are crossing of leads during recording, especially arm leads, mislabeling of leads, overdamping of the stylus, 60-cycle artifact, muscle tremor artifact, and a paper speed of 50 mm per second instead of 25. These may occur singly or in combination and may simulate or obscure heart disease. Technical error is discussed in Chapter XIV and suggestions are offered to help in its identification. To be really secure in this area, a doctor must have made tracings himself, and he must never underestimate or forget the importance of the technician.

STATEMENT OF THE INTERPRETATION

If information in the electrocardiogram is to be of the greatest

ST		Example	T		Comment
J Displacement	Contour		Amplitude/Sign	Contour	
none	normal	1	usual/positive	normal	The range of normal is wide
up	normal	2	usual/positive	normal	This pattern is common as a "normal variant" called "early repolarization" but must be differentiated from the subepicardial injury of pericarditis and from early evidence of myocardial infarction
down	flattened	3	low/positive	not remarkable	Typical of subendocardial injury as with coronary insufficiency
none	sagging	4	low/positive	not remarkable	A common nonspecific abnormality
none	flattened	5	low/positive	not remarkable	A common nonspecific abnormality

proximal	contour		T amplitude	distal	Interpretation
up	arched	6	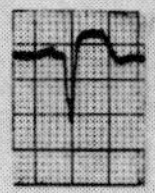 positive	inseparable from ST	Typical of myocardial injury and, when associated with QRS deformity of infarction, as it is here, evidence that the infarct is of recent origin (or that there is a ventricular aneurysm)
none	related to T	7	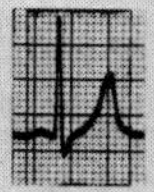 tall	symmetrical	Usually normal. Sometimes evidence of hyperkalemia, myocardial hypoxia, or intracranial lesion. Differential depends upon serial findings and the clinical setting
none	flattened	8	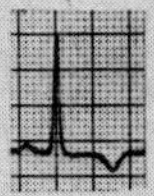 low/negative	symmetrical	This pattern in left chest leads may be nonspecific but often derives from discrepancy between supply of blood and demand for it and may be precipitated by left ventricular overload and/or coronary artery disease; symmetry favors the latter
none	normal	9	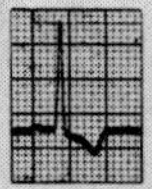 usual/negative	normal	The differential is similar to that immediately above. The normal contour of T is seen more commonly when left ventricular overload is the principal problem
none	related to T	10	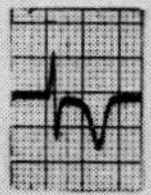 deep	symmetrical	Typical of myocardial hypoxia when transient and associated with chest pain. Common in mid-precordial leads. May be due to left ventricular overload and may be nonspecific

Figure 16-4. Description of ST-T complex. Information useful to the patient can come from identifying abnormality in the proximal part of the ST-T complex, ST displacement and contour, and the distal part, T amplitude and sign. Examples are given.

usefulness to the patient, the interpreter must know not only electrocardiography but also the clinical setting and what information the study is expected to yield. For him to arrive at a conclusion without this information would be like making a clinical diagnosis on the basis of physical examination without history; sometimes it is possible but it is never the best practice. It is all right for him to look at the tracing before knowing anything about the patient, as a matter of fact this should be routine in the interest of objectivity, and some abnormalities, such as disorders of mechanism, may be diagnosed without regard to the clinical problem, but before he reaches a conclusion and writes a report the electrocardiographer must consider all available information — and change his mind as often as necessary. *When there is doubt,* underinterpretation is better if the question is one of something that cannot be ruled in or out, a diagnosis that does not depend entirely upon the EKG and that might work to the patient's disadvantage, e.g., myocardial infarction, ventricular hypertrophy. If the implication is something that the doctor might not have thought about and that would help the patient without putting him at risk of harm, something that can be confirmed or excluded by other means, overinterpretation is justified, e.g., digitalis toxicity, electrolyte imbalance.

The statement of a clinical diagnosis incorporates three categories of information: topography, etiology, and manifestations. In not every case must each of these be identified individually, but the language used in writing the diagnosis should convey as much as possible about all of them to one familiar with the terminology and the method. A complete electrocardiographic interpretation informs in three categories, too — mechanism, structure, and function — and the level of confidence of each should be clear. It is meaningful to say that findings suggest an interpretation, or are typical or characteristic of one, or that a certain conclusion is probable, but caveats such as "possible" and "consistent with" diminish the value of the report, add nothing, and should be avoided. The interpretation should be as closely relevant as possible to topography, etiology, or symptoms and/or signs.

The tangible product of the electrocardiographer's practice is a message on a piece of paper to be used as an implement by another doctor in the care of his patient. The fact that the precision with which an EKG interpretation can be stated is limited by practical considerations, the realities of clinical medicine, and the way language is used and understood means that greater, not less, care must be taken in its preparation — and in its evaluation by the primary doctor.

REFERENCES

1. Wilson, F.N., Rosenbaum, F.F., and Johnston, F.D.: Interpretation of the ventricular complex of the electrocardiogram, Adv. Intern. Med., 2:1, 1947.
2. Harrison, T.R. (Ed.): Principles of Internal Medicine, Philadelphia and Toronto, Blakiston, 1950.
3. Bean, W.B.: The natural history of error, A.M.A., Arch. Intern. Med., 105:184, 1960.
4. Grant, R.P. (moderator): The electrocardiogram today: a symposium discussion, Am. J. Cardiol., 19:401, 1967.
5. Flowers, N.C., Horan, L.G., Tolleson, W.J., and Thomas, J.R.: Localization of the site of myocardial scarring in man by high frequency components, Circulation, 40:927, 1969.
6. Grant, R.P.: Architectronics of the heart, Am. Heart J., 46:405, 1953.
7. _____ The relationship between the anatomic position of the heart and the electrocardiogram. A criticism of "unipolar" electrocardiography, Circulation, 7:890, 1953.
8. Mathewson, F.A.L., and Varnam, G.S.: Abnormal electrocardiograms in apparently healthy people. I. Long-term follow-up study, Circulation, 21:196, 1960.
9. Johnston, F.D.: (Editorial): What is a normal electrocardiogram, Circulation, 24:707, 1961.
10. Smith, H.W.: Plato and Clementine, Bull. N.Y. Acad. Med., 23:352, 1947.
11. Epstein. F.H., Doyle, J.T., Pollack, A.A., Pollack, H., Robb, G.P., and Simonson, E.: Observer interpretation of electrocardiograms, J.A.M.A., 175:847, 1961.
12. Caceres, C.A.: A basis for observer variation in electrocardiographic interpretation, Prog. Cardiovasc. Dis., 5:521, 1963.
13. Levine, H.D.: Semantics and the electrocardiographic report, Am. Heart J., 65:433, 1963.
14. Grant's Clinical Electrocardiography, 2nd ed., Revised by Beckwith, J.R., New York, McGraw-Hill, Blakiston Division, 1970.
15. Hurst, J.W., and Myerburg, R.: Introduction to Electrocardiography, New York, McGraw-Hill, Blakiston Division, 1970.
16. Katz, L.N.: Electrocardiography, 2nd ed., Philadelphia, Lea & Febiger, 1946.

17. Lindsay, A.E., and Budkin, A.: The Cardiac Arrhythmias, Chicago, Year Book Medical Publishers, Inc., 1969.

18. Goldman, M.J.: Principles of Clinical Electrocardiography, 7th ed., Los Altos, Calif., Lange Medical Publications, 1970.

19. Lamb, L.E.: Electrocardiography and Vectorcardiography, Philadelphia and London, W.B. Saunders Company, 1965.

20. Hurst, J.W., and Logue, B.R. (Eds.): The Heart, 2nd ed., New York, McGraw-Hill, Blakiston Division, 1970.

21. Friedberg, C.K.: Diseases of the Heart, 3rd ed., Philadelphia and London, W.B. Saunders Company, 1966.

22. Harrison, T.R. (Ed.): Principles of Internal Medicine, 5th ed., New York, McGraw-Hill, Blakiston Division, 1966.

23. Burch, G.E., and DePasquale, N.P.: A History of Electrocardiography, Chicago, Year Book Medical Publishers, Inc., 1964.

24. Waller, A.D.: A Demonstration on man of electromotive changes accompanying the heart's beat, J. Physiol., 8:229, 1887.

25. Einthoven, W.: Die galvanometrische Registrirung des mensclichen Elektrokardiogramms zugleich eine Beurtheilung der Anwendung des Capillar-Elektrometers in der Physiologic, Arch. ges. Physiol. 99:472, 1903. Translated in: Classics of Cardiology, F.A. Willius, and T.E. Keys, Henry Schuman, Inc., Dover Publications, Inc., New York, 1961.

26. Einthoven, W.: Ueber die Form des menschlichen Electrocardiograms, Arch. ges. Physiol., 60:101, 1895. Quoted in Circ. Res., 22:220 (February) 1968.

27. Scherf, D.: Remarks on the nomenclature of cardiac arrhythmias, Progr. Cardiovasc. Dis., 13:1, 1970.

28. Wolferth, C.C., and Wood, F.C.: The electrocardiographic diagnosis of coronary occlusion by the use of chest leads, Am. J. Med. Sci., 183:30, 1932.

29. Wilson, F.N., MacLeod, A.B., and Barker, P.S.: Electrocardiographic leads which record potential variations produced by the heartbeat at a single point, Proc. Soc. Exp. Biol. Med., 29:1011, 1932.

30. Joint recommendations of the American Heart Association and the Cardiac Society of Great Britain and Ireland, a supplementary report. Standardization of precordial leads, Am. Heart J., 15:235, 1938.

31. Goldberger, E.: Unipolar Lead Electrocardiography and Vectrocardiography, 3rd ed., Philadelphia, Lea & Febiger, 1953.

32. Wilson, F.N., MacLeod, A.B., and Barker, P.A.: Electrocardiographic leads which record potential variations produced by the heartbeat at a single point, Proc. Soc. Exp. Biol. Med., 29:1011, 1932.

33. Sherf, L., and James, T.N.: A new electrocardiographic concept: synchronized sinoventricular conduction, Dis. Chest, 55:127, 1969.

34. Emberson, J.W., and Challice, C.E.: Studies on the impulse conducting pathways in the atrium of the mammalian heart, Am. Heart J., 79:653, 1970.

35. James, T.N.: The connecting pathways between the sinus node and AV node and between the right and the left atrium in the human heart, Am. Heart J., 66:498, 1963.

36. Scherf, D., and Cohen, J.: The Atrioventricular Node and Selected Cardiac Arrhythmias, New York, Grune and Stratton, 1964.

37. deCarvalho, A.P., deMello, W.C., and Hoffman, B.F. (Eds.): The Specialized Tissues of the Heart, Amsterdam, Elsevier, 1961.

38. James, T.N.: Morphology of the human atrioventricular node, with remarks pertinent to its electrophysiology, Am. Heart J., 62:756, 1961.

39. Surawicz, B.: Electrolytes and the electrocardiogram, Am. J. Cardiol., 12:656, 1963.

40. Hoffman B.F., and Cranefield, P.F.: Electrophysiology of the Heart, New York, McGraw-Hill, Blakiston Division, 1960.

41. Massumi, R.A., Sarin, R.K., Tawakkol, A.A., Rios, J.C., and Jackson, H.: Time sequence of right and left atrial depolarization as a guide to the origin of P waves, Am. J. Cardiol., 24:28, 1969.

42. Hoffman, B.F., Moore, E.N., Stuckey, J.H., and Cranefield, P.F.: Functional properties of the atrioventricular conduction system, Circ. Res., 13:308, 1963.

43. Medrano, G.A., DeMicheli, A., Cisneros, F., and Sodi-Pallares, D.: The anterior subdivision block of the left bundle branch of His. I. The ventricular activation process, J. Electrocardiol. 3:7, 1970.

44. Scher, A.M.: The general order of ventricular excitation. *In* Mechanisms and Therapy of Cardiac Arrhythmias, Dreifus, L.S., Likoff, W., and Moyer, J.H. (Eds.), New York and London, Grune and Stratton, 1966.

45. Fruehan, C.T., Baule, G., Burgess, M.J., Millar, K., and Abildskov, J.A.: Differences in the heart as a generator of the QRS and ST-T deflections, Am. Heart J., 77:842, 1969.

46. Christian, E., and Scher, A.M.: The effect of ventricular depolarization on the sequence of ventricular repolarization, Am. Heart J., 74:530, 1967.

47. Crain, B., Burgess, M.J., Millar, K., and Abildskov, J.A.: Observations concerning the validity of the ventricular gradient concept, Am. Heart J., 78:796, 1969.

48. Abildskov, J.A., Burgess, M.J., Millar, K., and Wyatt, R.: New data and concepts concerning the ventricular gradient, Chest, 58:244, 1970.

49. Simonson, E., Schmitt, O.H., Dahl, J., Fry, D., and Bakken, E.E.: The theoretical and experimental bases of the frontal plane ventric-

ular gradient and its spatial counterpart, Am. Heart J., 47:122, 1954.

50. Millar, K., Burgess, M.J., and Abildskov, J.A.: Influence of activation order on QRST area, Circulation, 42-111:98, 1970.

51. Lepeschkin, E.: The U wave of the electrocardiogram: a symposium, Circulation, 15:68, 1957.

52. ____ The U wave of the electrocardiogram, Mod. Con. Cardiovasc. Dis., 38:39, 1969.

53. Blake, T.M.: The question of axis deviation, Southern Med. J., 60:1110, 1967.

54. Stinebaugh, B.J., Schloeder, F.X., and DeAlba, E.: An evaluation of the frontal plane QRS-T angle in normal adults, Arch. Intern. Med., 116:810, 1965.

55. Burch, G.E., DePasquale, N.P., and Cronvich, J.A.: A standard reference system for spatial vectorcardiography. Comparison of the equilateral tetrahedron and Frank systems, Am. Heart J., 80:638, 1970.

56. ____ Abildskov, J.A., and Cronvich, J.A.: Studies of the spatial vectorcardiogram in normal man, Circulation, 7:558, 1953.

57. Mirowski, M.: Ectopic rhythms originating anteriorly in the left atrium. Am. Heart J., 74:299, 1967.

58. McCaughan, D., Primeau, R.E., and Littmann, D.: The precordial T wave, Am. J. Cardiol., 20:660, 1967.

59. Abildskov, J.A., and Wilkinson, Jr., R.S.: The relation of precordial and orthogonal leads, Circulation, 27:58, 1963.

60. Herbert, W.H., and Sobol, B.J.: Normal atrioventricular conduction time, Am. J. Med., 48:145, 1970.

61. Lepeschkin, E., and Surawicz, B.: The measurement of the duration of the QRS interval, Am. Heart J., 44:80, 1952.

62. Susmano, A., Graettinger, J.S., and Carleton, R.A.: The relationship between QT intrval and heart rate, Electrocardiology, 2:269, 1969.

63. Simonson, E.: QRS-T angle at various ages, Circulation, 14:100, 1956.

64. Stinebaugh, B.J., Schloeder, F.X., and DeAlba, E.: An evaluation of the frontal plane QRS-T angle in normal adults, Arch. Intern. Med., 116:810, 1965.

65. Ziegler, R., and Bloomfield, D.K.: A study of the normal QRS-T angle in the frontal plane, J. Electrocardiol., 3:161, 1970.

66. Hoffman, B.F.: Physiologic basis of disturbances of cardiac rhythm and conduction, Prog. Cardiovasc. Dis., 2:319, 1959.

67. Scherf, D.: The mechanism of sinoatrial block, Am. J. Cardiol., 23:769, 1969.

68. Greenwood, R.J., and Finkelstein, D.: Sinoatrial Heart Block, Springfield, Ill., Charles C Thomas, 1964.

69. Prinzmetal, M., Corday, E., Brill, I.C., Oblath, R.W., and Kruger, H.E.: The Auricular Arrhythmias, Springfield, Ill., Charles C Thomas, 1952.

70. Scherf, D.: Mechanism of atrial flutter and fibrillation, *In* Mechanisms and Therapy of Cardiac Arrhythmias, Dreifus, L.S., Likoff, W., and Moyer, J.H. (Eds.), New York, Grune and Stratton, 1966.

71. Wallace, A.G., and Daggett, W.M.: Re-excitation of the atrium. "The echo phenomenon," Am. Heart J., 68:661, 1964.

72. Han, J.: The mechanism of paroxysmal atrial tachycardia, sustained reciprocation, Am. J. Cardiol., 26:329, 1970.

73. Bigger, Jr., J.T., and Goldreyer, B.N.: The mechanism of supraventricular tachycardia, Circulation, 42:673, 1970.

74. Choen, J., and Scherf, D.: Complete interatrial and intra-atrial block (atrial dissociation), Am. Heart J., 70:23, 1965.

75. Steffens, T.G.: A report of atrial parasystole. J. Electrocardiol., 3:177, 1970.

76. Wit, A.L., Damato, A.N., Weill, M.B., and Steiner, C.: Phenomenon of the gap in atrioventricular conduction in the human heart. Circ. Res., 27:679, 1970.

77. Rodensky, P.L., and Wasserman, F.: Atrial flutter with 1:1 conduction, Dis. Chest, 38:563, 1960.

78. Shine, K.I., Kastor, J.A., and Yurchak, P.M.: Multifocal atrial tachycardia: clinical and electrocardiographic features, N. Engl. J. Med., 279:344, 1968.

79. Lipson, M.J., and Naimi, Shapur: Multifocal atrial tachycardia (chaotic atrial tachycardia): clinical association and significance, Circulation, 42:397, 1970.

80. Rosner, S.W.: Atrial tachysystole with block, Circulation, 29:614, 1964.

81. Lown, B., and Levine, H.D.: Atrial Arrhythmias, Digitalis, and Potassium, New York, Landsberger Medical Books, Inc., 1952.

82. Mark, Herbert, and Sham, R.: Nondigitalis induced paroxysmal atrial tachycardia with block. I. Management with cardioversion, J. Electrocardiol., 2:171, 1969.

83. Moore, E.N., and Melbin, J.: Experimental studies on buried P waves, J. Electrocardiol., 3:1, 1970.

84. Chung, Edward K.: Atrial dissociation due to unilateral atrial fibrillation, J. Electrocardiol., 2:373, 1969.

85. Hoffman, B.F., and Cranefield, P.F.: The physiologic basis of cardiac arrhythmias, Am. J.Med., 37:670, 1964.

86. Massumi, R.A.: Interpolated His bundle extrasystoles. An unusual cause of tachycardia, Am. J. Med., 49:265, 1970.

87. Marriot, H.J.L., and Bradley, S.M.: Main-stem extrasystoles, Cir-

culation, 16:544, 1957.

88. Massumi, R., and Tawakkol, A.A.: Direct study of left atrial P waves, Am. J. Cardiol., 20:331, 1967.

89. Harris, B.C., Shaver, J.A., Gray, III, S., Kroetz, F.W., and Leonard, J.J.: Left atrial rhythm; experimental production in man, Circulation, 37:1000, 1968.

90. Frankel, W.S., and Soloff, L.A.: Left atrial rhythm: analysis by intra-atrial electrocardiogram and the vectorcardiogram, Am. J. Cardiol., 22:645, 1968.

91. Lau, S.H., Cohen, S.I., Stein, E., Haft, J.I., Rose, K.M., and Damato, A.N.: P waves and P loops in coronary sinus and left atrial ectopic rhythms, Am. Heart J., 79:201, 1970.

92. Leon, D.F., Lancster, J.F., Shaver, J.A., Kroetz, F.W., and Leonard, J.J.: Right atrial ectopic rhythms. Experimental production in man, Am. J. Cardiol., 25:6, 1970.

93. Mirowski, M., Lau, S.H., Bobb, G.A., Steiner, C., and Damato, A.N.: Studies on left atrial automaticity in dogs, Circ. Res., 26:317, 1970.

94. Piccolo, E., Nava, A., Furlanello, F., Permutti, B., and Dalla Volta, D.: Left atrial rhythm. Vectorcardiographic study and electrophysio-logic critical evaluation, Am. Heart J., 80:11, 1970.

95. Waldo, A.L., Vitikainen, K.J., Kaiser, G.A., Malm, J.R., and Hoff-man, B.F.: The P wave and PR interval: effects of the site of origin of atrial depolarization, Circulation, 42:653, 1970.

96. Damato, A.N., and Lau, S.H.: His bundle rhythm, Circulation, 40:527, 1969.

97. Fisch, C., and Knoebel, S.B.: Junctional rhythms, Prog. Cardiovasc. Dis., 13:141, 1970.

98. Mirowski, M., and Tabatznik, B.: The spatial characteristics of atrial activation in ventriculoatrial excitation, Chest, 57:9, 1970.

99. Marriott, H.L.L.: Retrograde doubts, Chest, 57:2, 1970.

100. Castellanos, Jr., A., Castillo, C., and Lemberg, L.: His bundle electrocardiography: A programmed introduction, Chest, 57:350, 1970.

101. Damato, A.N., and Lau, S.H.: Clinical value of the electrogram of the conduction system, Prog. Cardiovasc. Dis., 13:119, 1970.

102. Patton, R.D., Stein, E., Rosen, K.M., Lau, S.H., and Damato, A.N.: Bundle of His electrograms: a new method for analyzing arrhyth-mias, Am. J. Cardiol., 26:324, 1970.

103. Cohen, S.I., Lau, S.H., Berkowitz, W.D., and Damato, A.N.: Con-cealed conduction during atrial fibrillation, Am. J. Cardiol., 25:416, 1970.

104. Massumi, R.A., and Ali, N.: Accelerated isorhythmic ventricular rhythms, Am. J. Cardiol., 26:170, 1970.

105. Langendorf, R.: Concealed AV conduction: the effect of blocked impulses on the formation and conduction of subsequent impulses, Am. Heart J, 35:542, 1948.

106. Kastor, J.A., and Yurchak, P.M.: Recognition of digitalis intoxication in the presence of atrial fibrillation, Ann. Intern. Med., 67:1045, 1967.

107. Javier, R.P., Narula, O.S., and Samet, P.: Atrial tachysystole (flutter?) with apparent exit block, Circulation, 40:179, 1969.

108. Pick, A.: Electrocardiographic features of exit-block. *In* Mechanisms and Therapy of Cardiac Arrhythmias, Dreifus, L.S., Likoff, W., and Moyer, J.H. (Eds.), New York, Grune and Stratton, Inc., 469, 1966.

109. Damato, A.N., Lau, S.H., and Bobb, G.A.: Studies on ventriculo-atrial conduction and the re-entry phenomenon, Circulation, 41:423, 1970.

110. Goldreyer, B.N., and Bigger, Jr., J.T.: Ventriculo-atrial conduction in man, Circulation, 41:935, 1970.

111. Moe, G.K., Mendez, C., and Han, J.: Some features of a dual A-V conduction system. *In* Mechanisms and Therapy of Cardiac Arrhythmias, Dreifus, L.S., Likoff, W., and Moyer, J.H. (Eds.), New York, Grune and Stratton, 361, 1966.

112. Wit, A.L., Weiss, M.B., Berkowitz, W.D., Rosen, K.M., Steiner, C., and Damato, A.N.: Patterns of atrioventricular conduction in the human heart, Circ. Res., 27:345, 1970.

113. Roelandt, J., and Van der Hauwaert, L.: Atrial reciprocal rhythm and reciprocating tachycardia in Wolff-Parkinson-White syndrome, Circulation, 38:64, 1968.

114. Schamroth, L., and Yoshonis, K.F.: Mechanisms in reciprocal rhythm, Am. J. Cardiol., 24:224, 1969.

115. Han, J.: The mechanism of paroxysmal atrial tachycardial. Sustained reciprocation, Am. J. Cardiol., 26:329, 1970.

116. Gulotta, S.J., and Aronson, A.L.: Cardioversion of atrial tachycardia and flutter by atrial stimulation. Am. J. Cardiol., 26:262, 1970.

117. Schuilenburg, R.M., and Durrer, D.: Atrial echo beats in the human heart induced by atrial premature beats, Circulation, 37:680, 1968.

118. _____ and Durrer, D.: Ventricular echo beats in the human heart elicited by induced ventricular premature beats, Circulation, 40:337, 1969.

119. Moe, G.K., Childers, R.W., and Meredith, J.: An appraisal of "supernormal" AV conduction, Circulation, 38:5, 1968.

120. Mihalick, M., and Fisch, C.: Supernormal conduction of the right bundle branch, Chest, 57:395, 1970.

121. Pick, A., Langendorf, R., and Katz, L.N.: The supernormal phase of atrioventricular conduction. I. Fundamental mechanisms, Circulation, 26:388, 1962.

122. Soloff, L.A., and Fewell, J.W.: The supernormal phase of ventricular conduction in man. Its bearing on the genesis of ventricular premature systoles, and a note of atrioventricular conduction, Am. Heart J., 59:869, 1960.

123. Rosenbaum, M.B.: Classification of ventricular extrasystoles according to form, J. Electrocardiol., 2:289, 1969.

124. Killip, T.: Dysrhythmia prophylaxis, N. Engl. J. Med., 281:1304, 1969.

125. Massumi, R.A., Tawakkol, A.A., and Kistin, A.D.: Re-evaluation of electrocardiographic and bedside criteria for diagnosis of ventricular tachycardia, Circulation, 36:628, 1967.

126. Hair, J., Thomas, E., Eagan, J.T., and Orgain, E.S.: Paroxysmal ventricular tachycardia in the absence of demonstrable heart disease, Am. J. Cardiol., 9:209, 1962.

127. Rosenbaum, M.B., Elizari, M.V., and Lazzari, J.O.: The mechanism of bidirectional tachycardia, Am. Heart J., 78:4, 1969.

128. Ledwich, J.R., and Fay, J.E.: Idiopathic recurrent ventricular fibrillation, Am. J. Cardiol., 24:255, 1969.

129. Wild, J.B., and Grover, J.D.: The fist as an external cardiac pacemaker, Lancet, II:436, 1970.

130. Armbrust, Jr., C.A., and Levine, S.A.: Paroxysmal ventricular tachycardia: a study of a hundred and seven cases, Circulation, 1:28, 1950.

131. Herrmann, G.R., Park, H.M., and Hejtmancik, M.R.: Paroxysmal ventricular tachycardia: a clinical and electrocardiographic study, Am. Heart J., 57:166, 1959.

132. Castellanos, Jr., A., Lemberg, L., and Arcebal, A.G.: Mechanisms of slow ventricular tachycardias in acute myocardial infarction, Dis. Chest, 56:470, 1969.

133. Dishpande, S.Y., and Magendantz, H.H.: AV nodal parasystole associated with complete AV block, Am. J. Cardiol., 23:98, 1969.

134. Scherf, D., Blumenfield, S., and Yildoz, M.: Extrasystoles and parasystole, Am. Heart J., 64:357, 1962.

135. Chung, E.K.Y.: Parasystole, Prog. Cardiovasc. Dis., 11:64, 1968.

136. Narula, O.S., and Samet, P.: Wenckebach and Mobitz type II AV block due to block within the His bundle and bundle branches, Circulation, 41:947, 1970.

137. Rosselot, E., Ahumanda, J., Spoererl, A., and Sepulveda, G.: Trifascicular block treated by artificial pacing, Am. J. Cardiol., 26:6, 1970.

138. Harper, J.R., Harley, A., Hackel, D.B., Estes, Jr., E.H.: Coronary artery disease and major conduction disturbances, Am. Heart J., 77:411, 1969.

139. Wenckebach, K.F.: Zur Analyse des urregelmassingen Pulses, Z. Klin. Med., 37:475, 1899.

140. Hay, J.: Bradycardia and cardiac arrhythmia produced by depression of certain of the functions of the heart, Lancet, I:139, 1906.

141. Mobitz, W.: Uber de unvollstandige Storung der Erregungstuber-leitung zwischen Vorhof und Kammer des manschlichen Herzens, Z. Ges. Exp. Med., 41:180, 1924.

142. Schaffer, A.I.: Mechanism of Wenckebach type of atrioventricular block, Am. Heart J., 79:138, 1970.

143. Langendorf, R., and Pick, A.: Atrioventricular block, Type II (Mobitz) — its nature and clinical significance, Circulation, 38:819, 1968.

144. Rosenbaum, M.B., and Lepeschkin, E.: Bilateral bundle branch block, Am. Heart J., 50:38, 1955.

145. Schluger, J., Iraj, I., and Edson, J.N.: Cardiac pacing in acute myocardial infarction complicated by complete heart block, Am. Heart J., 80:116, 1970.

146. Brown, R.W., Hunt, D., and Sloman, J.G.: The natural history of atrioventricular conduction defects in acute myocardial infarction, Am. Heart J., 78:460, 1969.

147. Feldt, R.H., DuShane, J.W., and Titus, J.L.: The atrioventricular conduction system in persistent common atrioventricular canal defect: correlations with electrocardiogram, Circulation, 42:437, 1970.

148. Wild, J.B., and Grover, J.D.: The fist as an external cardiac pace-maker, Lancet, II;436, 1970.

149. Rosenbaum, M.B.: Types of right bundle branch block and their clinical significance, J. Electrocardiol., 1:221, 1968.

150. ——— Elizari, M.V., Lazzari, J.O., Nau, G.G., Levi, R.J., and Hal-pern, M.S.: Intraventricular trifascicular blocks. The syndrome of right bundle branch block with intermittent left anterior and posterior hemiblock, Am. Heart J., 78:306, 1969.

151. ——— Intraventricular trifascicular blocks. Review of the literature and classification, Am. Heart J., 78:450, 1969.

152. Supulveda, G., Rosselot, E., and Ahumanda, J.: Second degree atrio-ventricular block with intermittent right plus left anterior branch block, Dis. Chest, 56:553, 1969.

153. Phibbs, B.: Interference, dissociation, and semantics. A plea for rational nomenclature, Am. Heart J., 65:283, 1963.

154. Pick, A.: A-V Dissociation. A proposal for a comprehensive clas-sification and consistent terminology, Am. Heart J., 66:147, 1963.

155. Mariott, H.J.L., and Menendez, M.M.: A-V dissociation revisited, Prog. Cardiovasc. Dis., 8:522, 1966.

156. Leighton, R.F., Ryan, J.M., Goodwin, R.S., Wooley, C.F., and Wesslen, A.M.: Incomplete left bundle branch block: the view from transseptal intraventricular leads, Circulation, 36:261, 1967.

157. Unger, P.N., Greenblatt, M., and Lev, M.: The anatomic basis of the electrocardiographic abnormality in incomplete left bundle branch block, Am. Heart J., 76:486, 1968.

158. Barold, S.S., Linhart, J.W., Hildner, F.J., Narula, O.S., and Lancaster, M.C.: Incomlete left bundle branch block: a definite electrocardiographic entity, Circulation, 38:702, 1968.

159. Grant, R.P.: Left axis deviation: an electrocardiographic-pathologic correlation study, Circulation, 14:233, 1956.

160. Pryor, R., and Blount, S.G.: The clinical significance of true left axis deviation. Left intraventricular blocks, Am. Heart J., 72:391, 1966.

161. Watt, T.B., Murao, S., and Pruitt, R.D.: Left axis deviation induced experimentally in a primate heart, Am. Heart J., 70:381, 1965.

162. Rosenbaum, M.B.: Types of left bundle branch block and their significance, J. Electrocardiol., 2:197, 1969.

163. ____ Elizari, M.V., Levi, R.J., Nau, G.J., Pisani, N., Lazzari, J.O., and Halpern, M.S.: Five cases of intermittent left anterior hemiblock, Am. J. Cardiol., 24:1, 1969.

164. ____ Elizari, M.V., and Lazzari, J.O.: The Hemiblocks, Oldsmar, Florida, Tampa Tracings, 1970.

165. Castellanos, Jr., A., Maytin, O., Arcebal, A.G., and Lemberg, L.: Alternating and coexisting block in the divisions of the left bundle branch, Dis. Chest, 56:103, 1969.

166. Castellanos, Jr., A., Lemberg, L., Arcebal, A.G., and Claxton, B.W.: Post-infarction conduction disturbances: a self-teaching program, Dis. Chest, 56:421, 1969.

167. Fernandez, F., Scebat, L., and Lenegre, J.: Electrocardiographic study of left intraventricular hemiblock in man during selective coronary arteriography, Am. J. Cardiol., 26:1, 1970.

168. Mariott, H.J.L., and Hogan, P.: Hemiblock in acute myocardial infarction, Chest, 58:342, 1970.

169. Watt, Jr., T.B., and Pruitt, R.: Left posterior fascicular block in canine and primate hearts: an electrocardiographic study, Circulation, 40:677, 1969.

170. Rosenbaum, M.B.: Types of left bundle branch block and their clinical significance, J. Electrocardiol., 2:197, 1969.

171. Castellanos, Jr., A., Maytin, O., Arcebal, A.G., and Lemberg, L.: Significance of complete right bundle branch block with right axis deviation in absence of right ventricular hypertrophy, Br. Heart J., 32:85, 1970.

172. Dodge, H.T., and Grant, R.P.: Mechanisms of QRS prolongation in man. Right ventricular conduction defects, Am. J. Med., 21:534, 1956.

173. Lasser, R.P., Haft, J.I., and Freidberg, C.K.: Relationship of right bundle branch block and marked left axis deviation (with left parietal

or peri-infarction block) to complete heart block and syncope, Circulation, 37:429, 1968.

174. Watt, Jr., T.B., and Pruitt, R.D.: Character, cause, and consequence of combined left axis deviation and right bundle branch block in human electrocardiograms, Am. Heart J., 77:460, 1969.

175. Rothfield, E.L., Zucker, I.R., Tiu, R., and Parsonnet, V.: The electrocardiographic syndrome of superior axis and right bundle branch block, Dis. Chest, 55:306, 1969.

176. Godman, M.J., Lassers, B.W., and Julian, D.G.: Complete bundle branch block complicating acute myocardial infarction, N. Engl. J. Med., 282:237, 1970.

177. Schuilenburg, R.M., and Durrer, D.: Observations on atrioventricular conduction in patients with bilateral bundle branch block, Circulation, 41:967, 1970.

178. Narula, O.S., Javier, R.P., Samet, P., and Maramba, L.C.: Significance of His and left bundle recordings from the left heart in man, Circulation, 42:385, 1970.

179. Wolff, L., Parkinson, J., and White, P.D.: Bundle branch block with short PR interval in healthy young people prone to paroxysmal tachycardia, Am. Heart J., 5:685, 1930.

180. _____ Wolff-Parkinson-White syndrome: historical and clinical features, Prog. Cardiovasc. Dis., 2:677, 1959.

181. Ferrer, I.: New concepts relating to the pre-excitation syndrome, J.A.M.A., 201:1038, 1967.

182. James, T.N.: The Wolff-Parkinson-White syndrome, Ann. Intern. Med., 71:339, 1969.

183. Durrer, D., Schuilenburg, R.M., and Wellens, H.J.J.: Pre-excitation revisited, Am. J. Cardiol., 25:690, 1970.

184. James, T.N.: The Wolff-Parkinson-White syndrome: evolving concepts of its pathogenesis, Prog. Cardiovasc. Dis., 13:159, 1970.

185. Hejtmancik, M.R., and Herrmann, G.R.: The electrocardiographic syndrome of short PR interval and broad QRS complexes, Am. Heart J., 54:708, 1957.

186. Berkman, N.L., and Lamb, L.E.: Wolff-Parkinson-White electrocardiogram: follow-up of five to twenty-eight years, N. Engl. J. Med., 278:492, 1968.

187. Castellanos, Jr., A., Mayer, J.W., and Lemberg, L.: The electrocardiogram and vectorcardiogram in Wolff-Parkinson-White syndrome associated with bundle branch block, Am. J. Cardiol., 10:657, 1962.

188. Marriott, H.J.L., and Rogers, H.M.: Mimics of ventricular tachycardia associated with the W-P-W syndrome, J. Electrocardiol., 2:77, 1969.

189. Wasserburger, R.H., White, D.H., and Lindsay, E.R.: Noninfarc-

tional QS$_{2,3}$, and aVF complexes as seen in the Wolff-Parkinson-White syndrome and left bundle branch block, Am. Heart J., 64:617, 1962.

190. Thomas, J.R.: Sequential ECG changes in myocardial infarction in the W-P-W syndrome, Dis. Chest, 53:217, 1968.

191. Kulbertus, H.E., and Collignon, P.G.: Ventricular pre-excitation simulating anteroseptal infarction, Dis. Chest, 56:461, 1969.

192. Sodi-Pallares, D., Cisneros, F., Medrano, G.A., Bisteni, A., Testelli, M.R., and deMicheli, A.: Electrocardiographic diagnosis of myocardial infarction in the presence of bundle branch block (right and left), ventricular premature beats and Wolff-Parkinson-White syndrome, Prog. Cardiovasc. Dis., 6:107, 1963.

193. Cole, J.S., Wills, R.E., Winterschied, L.C., Reichenbach, D.D., and Blackmon, J.R.: The Wolff-Parkinson-White syndrome: problems in evaluation and surgical therapy, Circulation, 42:111, 1970.

194. Cobb, F.R., Blumenschein, S.D., Sealy, W.C., et al. Successful surgical interruption of the bundle of Kent in a patient with Wolff-Parkinson-White syndrome, Circulation, 38:1018, 1968.

195. Entman, M.L., Estes, Jr., E.H., and Hackel, D.B.: The pathologic basis of the electrocardiographic pattern of parietal block, Am. Heart J., 74:202, 1967.

196. Corne, R.A., Parkin, T.W., Brandenburg, R.O., and Brown, Jr., A.L.: Peri-infarction block: postmyocardial-infarction intraventricular conduction disturbance, Am. Heart J., 69:150, 1965.

197. Castle, C.H., and Keane, W.M.: Electrocardiographic "peri-infarction block." A clinical and pathologic correlation, Circulation, 33:403, 1965.

198. Grant, R.P.: Peri-infarction block, Prog. Cardiovasc. Dis., 2:237, 1959.

199. Marriott, H.J.L.: Simulation of ectopic ventricular mechanisms, J.A.M.A., 196:787, 1966.

200. Cohen, S.I., Lau, S.H., Haft, J.I., and Damato, A.N.: Experimental production of aberrant ventricular conduction in man, Circulation, 36:673, 1967.

201. _____ Lau, S.H., Stein, E., Young, M.W., and Damato, A.D.: Variations of aberrant ventricular conduction in man: evidence of isolated and combined block within the specialized conduction system: and electrocardiographic and vectorcardiographic study, Circulation, 38:899, 1968.

202. Parameswaran, R., Monheit, R., and Goldberg, H.: Aberrant conduction due to retrograde activation of the right bundle branch, J. Electrocardiol., 3:173, 1970.

203. Surawicz, B., and Lasseter, K.L.: Effect of drugs on the electrocardiogram, Prog. Cardiovasc. Dis., 13:26, 1970.

204. Heissenbuttel, R.H., and Bigger, Jr., J.T.: The effect of oral quinidine on intraventricular conduction in man: correlation of plasma quinidine with changes in QRS duration, Am. Heart J., 80:453, 1970.

205. Jackson, D.H.: Transient post-traumatic right bundle branch block, Am. J. Cardiol., 23:877, 1969.

206. Lewis, C.M., Dagenais, G.R., Friesinger, G.C., and Ross, R.S.: Coronary aortographic appearances in patients with left bundle branch block, Circulation, 41:299, 1970.

207. Horan, L.G., Flowers, N.C., Tolleson, W.J., and Thomas, J.R.: The significance of diagnostic Q waves in the presence of bundle branch block, Chest, 58:214, 1970.

208. Walston, II, A., Boineau, J.P., Spach, M.S., Ayers, C.R., and Estes, Jr., E.H.: Relationship between ventricular depolarization and QRS in right and left bundle branch block, J. Electrocardiol., 1:155, 1968.

209. Booth, R.W., Chou, T.-C., and Scott, R.C.: Electrocardiographic diagnosis of ventricular hypertrophy in the presence of right bundle branch block, Circulation, 18:169, 1958.

210. Kossman, C.E., Burchell, H.B., Pruitt, R.D., and Scott, R.C.: The electrocardiogram in ventricular hypertrophy and bundle branch block. A panel discussion, Circulation, 26:1337, 1962.

211. Scott, R.C.: Left bundle branch block — a clinical assessment. Part III, Am. Heart J., 70:813, 1965.

212. Bauer, G.E.: Transient bundle branch block, Circulation, 29:730, 1964.

213. Krikler, D.M., and Lefevre, D.: Intermittent left bundle branch block without obvious heart disease, Lancet, I:498, 1970.

214. Gooch, A.S., and Crow, R.S.: Labile variations of intraventricular conduction unrelated to rate changes, Circulation, 38:480, 1968.

215. Massumi, R.A.: Bradycardia-dependent bundle branch block: a critique and proposed criteria, Circulation, 88:1066, 1968.

216. Sarachek, N.S.: Bradycardia-dependent bundle branch block. Relation to super-normal conduction and phase 4 depolarization, Am. J. Cardiol., 25:727, 1970.

217. Beach, I.B., Gracey, J.G., Peter, R.H., and Grunewald, P.W.: Benign left bundle branch block, Ann. Intern. Med., 70:269, 1969.

218. Bayley, R.H., and LaDue, J.S.: Electrocardiographic changes (local ventricular ischemia and injury), produced in the dog by temporary occlusion of a coronary artery, showing a new stage in the evolution of myocardial infarction, Am. Heart J., 27:164, 1944.

219. ____ and LaDue, J.S.: Electrocardiographic changes of impending infarction and the ischemia-injury pattern produced in the dog by total and subtotal occlusion of a coronary artery, Am. Heart J., 28:54, 1944.

220. Wasserburger, R.H., and Corliss, R.J.: Prominent precordial T

waves as an expression of coronary insufficiency, Am. J. Cardiol., 16:195, 1965.

221. Pinto, I.J., Nanda, N.C., Biswas, A.K., and Parulkar, V.G.: Tall, upright T waves in the precordial leads, Circulation, 36:708, 1967.

222. Grant, R.P., Estes, Jr., E.H., and Doyle, J.T.: Spatial vector electrocardiography. The clinical characteristics of ST and T vectors, Circulation, 3:182, 1951.

223. Caskey, T.D., and Estes, E.H.: Deviation of the ST segment. A review, Am. J. Med., 36:424, 1964.

224. Samson, W.E., and Scher, A.M.: Mechanism of ST segment alteration during acute myocardial injury, Circ. Res., 8:780, 1960.

225. Bishop, Jr., L.H., Estes, E.H., and McIntosh, H.D.: The electrocardiogram as a safeguard in pericardiocentesis, J.A.M.A., 162:264, 1956.

226. Boineau, J.P., Blumenschein, S., Spach, M.S., and Sabiston, D.C.: Relationship between ventricular depolarization and electrocardiogram in myocardial infarction, J. Electrocardiol., 1:233, 1968.

227. Durrer, D., Van Lier, A.A.W., and Buller, J.: Epicardial and intramural excitation in chronic myocardial infarction, Am. Heart J., 68:765, 1964.

228. Maxwell, M., Kennamer, R., and Prinzemetal, M.: Studies on the mechanism of ventricular activity. IX. The "mural type" coronary QS wave, Am. J. Med., 17:614, 1954.

229. Grant, R.P., and Murray, R.H.: The QRS complex deformity of myocardial infarction in the human subject, Am. J. Med., 17:587, 1954.

230. Perloff, J.K.: The recognition of strictly posterior myocardial infarction by conventional scalar electrocardiography, Circulation, 30:706, 1964.

231. Zakopoulos, K.S., and Tsatas, A.T.: Old "strictly posterior" myocardial infarction, Dis. Chest, 49:545, 1966.

232. Myers, G.B., Klein, H.A., and Kiratzka, T.: Correlation of electrocardiographic and pathologic findings in large anterolateral infarcts, Am. Heart J., 36:838, 1948.

233. Paton, B.C.: The accuracy of diagnosis of myocardial infarction. A clinicopathologic study, Am. J. Med., 23:761, 1957.

234. Wood, J.D., Laurie, W., and Smith, W.G.: The reliability of the electrocardiogram in myocardial infarction, Lancet, II:265, 1963.

235. Abbott, J., Scheinman, M., Schester, A., and Fleetwood, N.: Correlation of clinical and EKG changes in acute myocardial infarction, Circulation, 42-III:126, 1970.

236. Kaplan, B.M., and Berkson, D.M.: Serial electrocardiograms after myocardial infarction, Ann. Intern. Med., 60:430, 1964.

237. Burns-Cox, C.J.: Return to normal of the electrocardiogram after myocardial infarction, Lancet, I:1194, 1967.

238. _____ The occurrence of a normal electrocardiogram after myocardial infarction, Am. Heart J., 75:572, 1968.

239. Kalbfleisch, J.M., Shadaksharappa, K.S., Conrad, L.L., and Sarkar, N.K.: Disappearance of Q-deflection following myocardial infarction, Am. Heart J., 76:193, 1968.

240. Martinez-Rios, M.A., Bruto da Costa, B.C., Cecena-Seldner, F.A., and Gensini, G.G.: Normal electrocardiogram in the presence of severe coronary artery disease, Am. J. Cardiol., 25:320, 1970.

241. Fulton, M.C., and Marriott, H.J.L.: Acute pancreatitis simulating acute myocardial infarction in the electrocardiogram, Ann. Intern. Med., 59:730, 1963.

242. Ruskin, J., Whalen, R.E., and Orgain, E.S.: Electrocardiogram and vectorcardiogram simulating myocardial infarction in patient with pectus excavatum and straight back, Am. J. Cardiol., 21:446, 1968.

243. Penchas, S., and Keynan, A.: Acute myocardial infarction pattern in the ECG of a patient with funnel-chest, J. Electrocardiol., 2:285, 1969.

244. Pruitt, R.D., Curd, G.W., and Leachman, R.: Simulation of electrocardiogram of apicolateral myocardial infarction by myocardial destructive lesions of obscure etiology (myocardiopathy), Circulation, 25:506, 1962.

245. Hamby, R.I., and Raia, F.: Electrocardiographic aspects of primary myocardial disease in 60 patients, Am. Heart J., 76:316, 1968.

246. Tavel, M.E., and Fisch, C.: Abnormal Q waves simulating myocardial infarction in diffuse myocardial diseases, Am. Heart J., 68:534, 1964.

247. Lintermans, J.P., Kaplan, E.L., Morgan, B.C., Baum, D., and Guntheroth, W.G.: Infarction patterns in endocardial fibroelastosis, Circulation, 33:202, 1966.

248. Sodi-pallares, D., Bisteni, A., and Hermann, G.R.: Some views on the significance of qR and QR type complexes in right precordial leads in the absence of myocardial infarction, Am. Heart J., 43:716, 1952.

249. Gelzayd, E.A., and Holzman, D.: Electrocardiographic changes of hyperkalemia simulating acute myocardial infarction, Dis. Chest, 51:211, 1967.

250. Klein, H.O., Gross, H., and Rubin, I.L.: Transient electrocardiographic changes simulating myocardial infarction in open-heart surgery, Am. Heart J., 79:463, 1970.

251. Copeland, R.B., and Omenn, G.S.: Electrocardiogram changes suggestive of coronary artery disease in pneumothorax, Arch. Intern.

Med., 125:151, 1970.

252. Jones, Jr., F.L.: Transmural myocardial necrosis after nonpenetrating cardiac trauma, Am. J. Cardiol., 26:419, 1970.

253. Pruitt, R.D., Dennis, E.W., and Kinard, S.: The difficult electrocardiographic diagnosis of myocardial infarction, Prog. Cardiovasc. Dis., 6:85, 1963.

254. Mamlin, J.J., Weber, E.L., and Fisch, C.: Electrocardiographic pattern of massive myocardial infarction without pathologic confirmation, Circulation, 30:539, 1964.

255. Marriott, H.J.L.: Normal electrocardiographic variants simulating ischemic heart disease, J.A.M.A., 199:325, 1967.

256. Beamer, V., Amidi, M., and Scheuer, J.: Vectorcardiographic findings simulating myocardial infarction in aortic valve disease, J. Electrocardiol., 3:71, 1970.

257. Kini, P.M., Edelman, Jr., E.E., and Pipberger, H.V.: Electrocardiographic differentiation between left ventricular hypertrophy and anterior myocardial infarction, Circulation, 42:875, 1970.

258. Likoff, W., Segal, B., and Dreifus, L.: Myocardial infarction patterns in young subjects with normal coronary arteriogram, Circulation, 26:373, 1962.

259. Electrocardiographic infarction (editorial), J.A.M.A., 183:365, 1963.

260. Gross, H., Rubin, I.L., Lauffer, H., Bloomberg, A.E., Bujdoso, L., and Delman, A.J.: Transient abnormal Q waves in the dog without myocardial infarction, Am. J. Cardiol., 14:669, 1964.

261. Rubin, I.L., Gross, H., and Vigliano, E.M.: Transient abnormal Q waves during coronary insufficiency, Am. Heart J., 71:254, 1966.

262. Shugoll, G.I.: Transient QRS changes simulating myocardial infarction associated with shock and severe metabolic stress, Am. Heart J., 74:402, 1967.

263. Roesler, H., and Dressler, W.: Transient electrocardiographic changes identical with those of acute myocardial infarction accompanying attacks of angina pectoris, Am. Heart J., 47:520, 1954.

264. Phillips, J.H., DePasquale, N.P., and Burch, G.E.: The electrocardiogram in infarction of the anterolateral papillary muscle, Am. Heart J., 66:338, 1963.

265. Heikkila, J.: Electrocardiography in acute papillary muscle dysfunction and infarction: a clinicopathologic study, Chest, 57:510, 1970.

266. Sano, T., Ohshima, H., Fujita, T., Tsuchihashi, H., and Shimamoto, T.: Correlation of ECG, VCG, and pathologic findings in subendocardial infarcts and infarct-like lesions experimentally produced by administration of substances of high molecular weight, Am. Heart J., 62:167, 1961.

267. Georas, C.S., Dhalquist, E., and Cutts, F.B.: Subendocardial infarction; correlation of clinical, electrocardiographic, and pathologic data in 17 cases, Arch. Intern. Med., 111:488, 1963.

268. Salisbury, P., Cross, C.E., and Rieben, P.A.: Acute ischemia of inner layers of ventricular wall, Am. Heart J., 66:650, 1963.

269. Cook, R.W., Edwards, J.E., and Pruitt, R.D.: Electrocardiographic changes in acute subendocardial infarction. I. Large subendocardial and large nontransmural infarcts, Circulation, 18:603, 1958.

270. _____ Edwards, J.E., and Pruitt, R.D.: Electrocardiographic changes in acute subendocardial infarction. II. Small subendocardial infarcts, Circulations, 18:613, 1958.

271. Kostuk, W.J., and Beanlands, D.S.: Complete heart block associated with acute myocardial infarction, Am. J. Cardiol., 26:380, 1970.

272. Katz, K.H., Berk, M.S., and Mayman, C.H.: Acute myocardial infarction revealed in an isolated premature ventricular beat, Circulation, 18:897, 1958.

273. Benchimol, A.: Myocardial infarction and ectopic beats, J.A.M.A., 193:410, 1965.

274. Cohen, A.I.: Acute myocardial infarction revealed by interpolated premature ventricular contractions, Dis. Chest, 52:83, 1967.

275. Gedge, S.W., Achor, R.W.P., Berge, K.G., and Edwards, J.E.: Electrocardiographic and pathological study of clinically diagnosed multiple myocardial infarctions, Circulation, 32-11:13, 1965.

276. James, T.N.: Pathogenesis of arrhythmias in acute myocardial infarction, Am. J. Cardiol., 24:791, 1969.

277. Swan, H.J.C.: Pathogenesis of arrhythmias in myocardial infarction, Am. J. Cardiol., 24:836, 1969.

278. DePasquale, N.P.: The electrocardiogram in complicated acute myocardial infarction, Prog. Cardiovasc. Dis., 13:72, July 1970.

279. Moyer, J.B., and Hiller, G.I.: Cardiac aneurysm: clinical and electrocardiographic analysis, Am. Heart J., 41:340, 1951.

280. Flowers, N.C., and Horan, L.G.: Atrial infarction, Dis. Chest, 49:638, 1966.

281. Douglas, A.H.: Atrial infarction, Dis. Chest, 54:481, 1968.

282. Dicosky, C., and Zimmerman, H.A.: Atrial injury, J. Electrocardiol., 2:51, 1969.

283. Harris, T.R., Copeland, G.D., and Brady, D.A.: Progressive injury current with metastatic tumor of the heart. Case report and review of the literature, Am. Heart J., 69:392, 1965.

284. Langner, Jr., P.H.: Victims of the vector, Am. Heart J., 69:284, 1965.

285. Saha, N.C.: Study of the P wave in normal and obstructive lung disease in Delhi, Am. Heart J., 80:154, 1970.

286. Calatayud, J.B., Abad, J.M., Khoi, N.B., Stanbro, W.B., and Silver,

H.M.: P-wave changes in chronic obstructive pulmonary disease, Am. Heart J., 79:444, 1970.

287.   Morris, Jr., J.J., Estes, Jr., E.H., Whalen, R.E., Thompson, Jr., H.K., and McIntosh, H.D.: P wave analysis in valvular heart disease, Circulation, 29:242, 1964.

288.   Arevalo, A.C., Spagnuolo, M., and Feinstein, A.R.: EKG indication of left atrial enlargement, J.A.M.A., 185:358, 1963.

289.   Saunders, J.L., Calatayud, J.B., Shultz, K.J., Maranhao, V., Gooch, A.S., and Goldberg, H.: Evaluation of ECG criteria for P-wave abnormalities, Am. Heart J., 74:757, 1967.

290.   Kasser, I., and Kennedy, J.W.: The relationship of increased left atrial volume and pressure to abnormal P waves in the electrocardiogram, Circulation, 39:339, 1969.

291.   Human, G.P., and Snyman, H.W.: The value of the Macruz index in the diagnosis of atrial enlargement, Circulation, 27:935, 1963.

292.   Mathur, V.S., and Levine, H.D.: Vectorcardiographic differentiation between right ventricular hypertrophy and posterobasal myocardial infarction, Circulation, 42:883, 1970.

293.   Sokolow, M., and Lyon, T.P.: The ventricular complex in left ventricular hypertrophy as obtained by unipolar precordial and limb leads, Am. Heart J., 37:161, 1949.

294.   Blake, T.M., and Dear, H.D.: Electrocardiographic recognition of left overwork, Southern Med. J., 60:135, 1967.

295.   Causey, W.A., Felts, S.K., and Blake, T.M.: Electrocardiography in the evaluation of right ventricular overload, Southern Med. J., 62:166, 1969.

296.   Milnor, W.R.: Electrocardiogram and vectorcardiogram in right ventricular hypertrophy and right bundle branch block, Circulation, 16:348, 1957.

297.   Kannel, W.B., Gordon, T., and Offutt, D.: Left ventricular hypertrophy by electrocardiogram. Prevalance, incidence, and mortality in the Framingham study, Ann. Intern. Med., 71:89, 1969.

298.   Pagnoni, A., and Goodwin, J.F.: The cardiographic diagnosis of combined ventricular hypertrophy, Br. Heart J., 14:451, 1952.

299.   Kossman, C.E., Burchell, H.B., Pruitt, R.D., and Scott, R.C.: The electrocardiogram in ventricular hypertrophy and bundle branch block: a panel discussion, Circulation, 26:1337, 1962.

300.   Miquel, C., Sodi-Pallares, D., Cisneros, F., Pileggi, F., Medrano, G., and Bisteni, A.: Right bundle branch block and right ventricular hypertrophy: electrocardiographic and vectorcardiographic diagnosis, Am. J. Cardiol., 1:57, 1958.

301.   Scott, R.C., and Norris, R.J.: Electrocardiographic-pathologic correlation study of left ventricular hypertrophy in the presence of left bundle branch block, Circulation, 20:766, 1959.

302. Ostrander, L.D., and Weinstein, B.J.: Electrocardiographic changes after glucose ingestion, Circulation, 30:67, 1964.

303. Reynolds, E.W., and Tu, P.N.: Transmyocardial temperature gradient in dog and man: relation to the polarity of the T wave of the electrocardiogram, Circ. Res., 15:11, 1964.

304. Kemp, G.L., and Ellested, M.H.: The significance of hyperventilative and orthostatic T-wave changes on the electrocardiogram, Arch. Intern. Med., 121:518, 1968.

305. Mitchell, J.H., and Shapiro, A.D.: The relationship of adrenalin and T wave changes in anxiety state, Am. Heart J., 48:323, 1954.

306. Ostrander, Jr., L.D.: Relation of "silent" T wave inversion to cardiovascular disease in an epidemiologic study, Am. J. Cardiol., 25:325, 1970.

307. Lamb, L.E.: Electrocardiography and Vectorcardiography: Instrumentation, Fundamentals, and Clinical Application, Philadelphia and London, W.B. Saunders Company, 1965.

308. Black,an, N.S., and Kuskin, L.: Inverted T waves in the precordial electrocardiogram of normal adolescents, Am. Heart J., 67:304, 1964.

309. Wiener, L., Rios, J.C., and Massumi, R.A.: T wave inversion with elevated RS-T segment simulating myocardial injury, Am. Heart J., 67:684, 1964.

310. Rafailzadeh, M., Luria, M.H., Lochaya, S., and Sheffer, A.B.: Physiologic studies in a healthy adolescent with inverted precordial T waves, Dis. Chest, 52:101, 1967.

311. Chou, T.-C., Co, P., and Helm, R.A.: Vectorcardiographic analysis of T wave inversion in the right precordial leads, Am. Heart J., 78:75, 1969.

312. Wasserburger, R.H., and Alt, W.J.: The normal ST segment elevation variant, Am. J. Cardiol., 8:184, 1961.

313. Kuaity, J., Wexler, H., and Simonson, E.: The electrocardiographic ice water test, Am. Heart J., 77:569, 1969.

314. Kassebaum, D.G., Southerland, K.I., and Judkins, M.P.: A comparison of hypoxemic and exercise electrocardiography in coronary artery disease, Am. Heart J., 75:759, 1968.

315. O'Brien, K.P., Higgs, L.M., Glancy, D.L., et al.: Hemodynamic accompaniments of angina: a comparison during angina induced by exercise and by atrial pacing, Circulation, 39:735, 1969.

316. Parker, J.O., Chiong, M.A., West, R.O., and Case, R.B.: Sequential alterations in myocardial lactate metabolism, ST segments, and left ventricular function during angina induced by atrial pacing, Circulation, 40:113, 1969.

317. Simonson, E.: Use of the electrocardiogram in exercise tests, Am. Heart J., 66:552, 1963.

318. Master, A.M., and Rosenfeld, I.: Two-step exercise test: current status after twenty-five years, Mod. Con. Cardiovasc. Dis., 36:19, 1967.

319. ___ and Rosenfeld, I.: Exercise electrocardiography as an estimation of cardiac function, Dis. Chest, 51:347, 1967.

320. ___ The Master two-step test, Am. Heart J., 75:809, 1968.

321. ___ and Rosenfeld, I.: Current status of the two-step test, J. Electrocardiol., 1:5, 1968.

322. ___ The Master two-step test: some historical highlights and current concepts, S. C. Med. Assn., 65, Supplement 1:12, 1969.

323. ___ The "augmented" Master two-step test, Circulation, 42-111:19, 1970.

324. Rosenfeld, I., and Master, A.M.: Recording the electrocardiogram during the performance of the Master two-step test. II, Circulation, 29:212, 1964.

325. Lepeschkin, E., and Surawicz, B.: Characteristics of true-positive and false-positive resutls of electrocardiographic Master two-step tests, N. Engl. J. Med., 258:511, 1958.

326. Robb, G.P., and Marks, H.H.: Latent coronary artery disease. Determination of its presence and severity by the exercise electrocardiogram, Am. J. Cardiol., 13:603, 1964.

327. Master, A.M.: ST elevation, Am. Heart J., 80:434, 1970.

328. Fortuin, N.J., and Friesinger, G.C.: Exercise-induced ST segment elevation. Clinical, electrocardiographic, and arteriographic studies in twelve patients, Am. J.Med., 49:459, 1970.

329. Blackburn, H. and committee: The exercise electrocardiogram. Differences in interpretation. Report of a technical group on exercise electrocardiography, Am. J. Cardiol., 21:871, 1968.

330. Kawai, C., and Hultgran, H.N.: The effect of digitalis upon the exercise electrocardiogram, Am. Heart J., 68:409, 1964.

331. McHenry, P.L., Raia, F., and Apiado, O.: False positive ECG response to exercise secondary to hyperventilation: cineangiographic correlation, Am. Heart J., 79:683, 1970.

332. Gazes, P.C.: False-positive exercise test in the presence of Wolff-Parkinson-White syndrome, Am. Heart J., 78:13, 1969.

333. Beard, E.F., Garcia, E., Burke, G.E., and Dear, W.E.: Postexercise electrocardiogram in screening for latent ischemic heart disease, Dis. Chest, 56:405, 1969.

334. Datey, K.K., and Misra, S.N.: Evaluation of two-step exercise test in patients with heart disease of different etiologies, Dis. Chest, 53:294, 1968.

335. Rowell, L.B., Taylor, H.L., Simonson, E., and Carlson, W.S.: The physiologic fallacy of adjusting for body weight in performance of the

Master two-step test, Am. Heart J., 70:461, 1965.

336. Sheffied, L.T., and Reeves, T.J.: Graded exercise in the diagnosis of angina pectoris, Mod. Con. Cardiovasc. Dis., 34:1, 1965.

337. Doan, A.E., Peterson, D.R., Blackmon, J.R., and Bruce, R.A.: Myocardial ischemia after maximal exercise in healthy men: one year follow-up of physically active and inactive men, Am. J. Cardiol., 17:9, 1966.

338. Master, A.M.: Is the highest rate attained in the Master "two-step" test sufficient? Circulation, 42-111:19, 1970.

339. Goldbarg, A.N., Moran, J.F., and Resnekov, L.: Multistage electrocardiographic exercise tests. Principles and clinical applications, Am. J. Cardiol., 26:84, 1970.

340. Gutman, R.A., Alexander, E.R., Li, Y.-B., Chiang, B.-N., Watten, R.H., Ting, N., and Bruce, R.A.: Delay of ST depression after maximal exercise by walking for two minutes, Circulation, 42:229, 1970.

341. Fisch, C., and Knoebel, S.B.: Recognition and therapy of digitalis toxicity, Prog. Cardiovasc. Dis., 13:71, 1970.

342. Delman, A.J., and Stein, E.: Atrial flutter secondary to digitalis toxicity. Report of three cases and review of the literature, Circulation, 29:593, 1964.

343. Chung, E.K.: Digitalis-induced cardiac arrhythmias, Am. Heart J., 79:845, 1970.

344. Stern, S., and Eisenberg, S.: The effect of propranolol (Inderal) on the electrocardiogram of normal subjects, Am. Heart J., 77:192, 1969.

345. Rosen, K.M., Lau, S.H., Weiss, M.B., and Damato, A.N.: The effect of lidocaine on atrioventricular and intraventricular conduction in man, Am. J. Cardiol., 25:1, 1970.

346. Damato, A.N., Berkowitz, W.D., Patton, R.D., and Lau, S.H.: The effect of diphenylhydantoin on atrioventricular and intraventricular conduction in man, Am. Heart J., 79:51, 1970.

347. Sanghvi, L.M., and Mathur, B.B.: Electrocardiogram after chloroquine and emetine, Circulation, 32:281, 1965.

348. Schoonmaker, F.W., Osteen, R.T., and Greenfield, J.C.: Thioridazine (Mellaril)-induced ventricular tachycardia controlled with an artificial pacemaker, Ann. Intern. Med., 65:1076, 1966.

349. Surawicz, B.: Relationship between electrocardiogram and electrolytes, Am. Heart J., 73:814, 1967.

350. Merrill, A.J.: The significance of the electrocardiogram in electrolyte disturbances, Am. Heart J., 43:634, 1952.

351. Fletcher, G.F., Hurst, J.W., and Schlant, R.C.: Electrocardiographic changes in severe hypokalemia. A reappraisal, Am. J. Cardiol., 20:628, 1967.

352. Bronsky, D., Dubin, A., Waldstein, S., and Kushner, D.S.: Calcium and the electrocardiogram. I. The electrocardiographic manifestations of hypoparathyroidism, Am. J. Cardiol., 7:833, 1961.

353. ———— Dubin, A., Waldstein, S.S., and Kushner, D.S.: Calcium and the electrocardiogram. II. The electrocardiographic manifestations of hyperparathyroidism and of marked hypercalcemia from various other etiologies, Am. J. Cardiol., 7:883, 1961.

354. Reid, J.A., Enson, Y., Harvey, R.M., and Ferrer, M.I.: The effect of variations in blood pH upon the electrocardiogram in man, Circulation, 31:369, 1965.

355. Rohmilt, D., Susilavorn, B., and Chou, T.-C.: Unusual electrocardiographic manifestation of pulmonary embolism, Am. Heart J., 80:237, 1970.

356. Smith, McK., and Ray, C.T.: Electrocardiographic signs of early right ventricular enlargement in acute pulmonary embolism, Chest, 58:205, 1970.

357. Eliot, R.S., Millhon, W.A., and Millhon, J.: The clinical significance of marked uncomplicated left axis deviation in men without known disease, Am. J. Cardiol., 12:767, 1963.

358. Gorman, P.A., Calatayd, J.B., Abraham, S., and Caceres, C.A.: Effects of age and heart disease on the QRS axis during the seventh through the tenth decades, Am. Heart J., 67:39, 1964.

359. Gup, A.M., Franklin, R.B., and Hill, Jr., J.E.: The vectorcardiogram in children with left axis deviation and no apparent heart disease, Am. Heart J., 69:619, 1965.

360. Corne, R.A., Parkin, T.W., Brandenburg, R.O., and Brown, Jr., A.L.: Significance of marked left axis deviation. Electrocardiographic-pathologic correlative study, Am. J. Cardiol., 15:605, 1965.

361. Moller, J., Carlson, E., and Eliot, R.S.: Left axis deviation in children, Dis. Chest, 53:453, 1968.

362. Shirley, Jr., H., Davis, F., and Spano, J.: Value of the electrocardiogram in the diagnosis of intracranial disease, Dis. Chest, 53:223, 1968.

363. Falsetti, H.L., and Willson, R.L.: QRS voltage criteria for posterior unipolar chest leads in a normal population, Dis. Chest, 52:695, 1967.

364. Abildskov, J.A., Miller, K., Burgess, M.J., and Vincent, W.: The electrocardiogram and the central nervous system, Prog. Cardiovasc. Dis., 13:210, 1970.

365. Burch, G.E., Colcolough, H., and Giles, T.: Intracranial lesions and the heart, Am. Heart J., 80:574, 1970.

366. Dolara, A., Moranda, P., and Pampaloni, M.: Electrocardiographic findings in 98 consecutive nonpenetrating chest injuries, Dis. Chest, 52:50, 1967.

367. Zinsser, H.F., and Thind, G.S.: Right bundle branch block after non-penetrating injury to the chest wall., J.A.M.A., 207:1913, 1969.

368. Harris, L.K.: Transient right bundle branch block following blunt chest trauma, Am. J. Cardiol., 23:884, 1969.

369. Dolara, A., and Pozzi, L.: Atrioventricular and intraventricular conduction defects after nonpenetrating trauma, Am. Heart J., 72:138, 1966.

370. Castellanos, Jr., A., Ortiz, J.M., Pastis, N., and Castillo, C.: The electrocardiogram in patients with pacemakers, Prog. Cardiovasc. Dis., 13:190, 1970.

371. Levy, M.N., and Zieske, H.: Mechanism of synchronization in isorhythmic dissociation, Circ. Res., 27:429, 1970.

372. Garcia-Palmieri, M.R., Rodriguez, R.C., and Girod, C.: The electrocardiogram and vectorcardiogram in congenital heart disease, Am. Heart J., 68:556, 1964.

373. Sodi-Pallares, D. guest editor: Symposium on electrocardiography in congenital heart disease. Part I. Am. J. Cardiol., 21:617, 1968.

374. Daves, M.L., and Pryor, R.: Cardiac positions, Am. Heart J., 79:408, 1970.

375. Dower, G.E.: Some instrumental errors in electrocardiography, Circulation, 28:483, 1963.

376. Riseman, J.E.F., and Sagall, E.L.: Diagnostic problems resulting from improper electrocardiographic technique, J.A.M.A., 178:806, 1961.

377. Lepeschkin, E.: Electrocardiographic instrumentation, Prog. Cardiovasc. Dis., 5:498, 1963.

378. Geddes, L.A.: Where are today's pioneering manufacturers of electrocardiographs? J. Electrocardiol., 2:1, 1969.

379. Pipberger, H.V.: The "new" electrocardiographs: a step toward greater fidelity in recording, Circulation, 42:771, 1970.

380. Aronow, S., Bruner, J.M.R., Siegel, E.F., and Sloss, L.J.: Ventricular fibrillation associated with an electrically operated bed, N. Engl. J. Med., 28:31, 1969.

381. Berson, A.S., and Pipberger, H.V.: The low-frequency response of electrocardiographs, a frequent source of recording errors, Am. Heart J., 71:779, 1966.

382. Meyer, J.L.: Some instrument-induced errors in the electrocardiogram, J.A.M.A., 201:351, 1967.

383. Berson, A.S., and Pipberger, H.V.: Electrocardiographic distortions caused by inadequate high-frequency response of direct writing electrocardiographs, Am. Heart J., 74:208, 1967.

384. Hirschman, J.C., Baker, T.J., and Schiff, A.D.: Transoceanic radio transmission of electrocardiograms, Dis. Chest, 52:186, 1967.

385. Dobrow, R.J., Fieldman, A., Page, W., Clason, C., Gorman, P.A., Reinfrank, R.F., and Caceres, C.A.: Transmission of electrocardiograms from a community hospital for remote computer analysis, Am. J. Cardiol., 21:687, 1968.

386. Tabatznik, B., Mower, M.M., and Staewan, W.S.: Inexpensive presentation of prolonged electrocardiographic tape recordings, Am. Heart J., 74:377, 1967.

387. Caceres, C.A., and Hockberg, H.M.: Performance of the computer and physician in the analysis of the electrocardiogram, Am. Heart J., 79:439, 1970.

388. Friedberg, C.K.: Computers in cardiology, Prog. Cardiovasc. Dis., 13:86, 1970.

389. Gorman, P.A., and Evans, J.M.: Computer analysis of the electrocardiogram: evaluation of experience in a hospital heart station, Am. Heart J., 80:515, 1970.

390. Mattingly, R.F., and Larks, S.D.: The fetal electrocardiogram, J.A.M.A., 183:245, 1963.

391. Buxton, T.M., Hsu, I., and Barter, R.H.: Fetal electrocardiography, J.A.M.A., 185:441, 1963.

392. Hon, E.H.: The classification of fetal heart rate. I. A working classification, Obstet. Gynecol., 22:137, 1963.

393. Ferrer, M.I.: Instant electrocardiograms as a teaching aid, Dis. Chest, 56:344, 1969.

394. Robitaille, G.A., Phillips, J.H., Sumner, R.C., and Higgins, T.G.: The value of inspiratory leads in electrocardiographic diagnosis, Dis. Chest, 50:487, 1966.

395. Tranchesi, J., Adelardi, V., and de Oliveira, J.M.: Atrial repolarization — its importance in clinical electrocardiography, Circulation, 22:635, 1960.

396. Starmer, C.F., Whalen, R.E., and McIntosh, H.D.: Hazards of electric shock, Am. J. Cardiol., 14:537, 1964.

397. Watson, H.: Electrode catheters and the diagnostic application of electrocardiography in small children, Circulation, 29:284, 1964.

398. Spach, M.S., Silberberg, W.P., Boineau, J.P., Barr, R.C., Long, E.C., Gallie, T.M., Gabor, J.B., and Wallace, A.W.: Body surface isopotential maps in normal children, ages four to 14 years, Am. Heart J., 72:640, 1966.

399. Uhley, H.N.: Electrocardiographic telemetry from ambulances. A practical approach to mobile coronary care units, Am. Heart J., 80:838, 1970.

400. Spangler, R.D., Horman, M.J., Miller, S.W., Rotenberg, D.A., Birnholz, J.C., Simmons, R.L., Westura, E.E., and Fox, III, S.M.: A submaximal exercise electrocardiographic test as a method of detecting

occult ischemic heart disease, Am. Heart J., 80:752, 1970.

401. Smith, R.F., Jackson, D.H., Harthorne, J.W., and Sanders, C.A.: Acquired bundle branch block in a healthy population, Am. Heart J., 80:746, 1970.

402. Awa, S., Linde, L.M., Oshima, M., Okuni, M., Momma, K., and Kakamura, N.: The significance of late-phased dart T wave in the electrocardiogram of children, Am. Heart J., 80:619, 1970.

403. Cabrera, E., and Gaxiola, A.: A critical re-evaluation of systolic and diastolic overloading patterns, Prog. Cardiovasc. Dis., 2:219, 1959.

404. Kastor, J.A., and Leinbach, R.C.: Pacemakers and their arrhythmias, Prog. Cardiovasc. Dis., 13:240, 1970.

405. Guy, C., and Eliot, R.S.: The subendocardium of the left ventricle, a physiologic enigma, Chest, 58:555, 1970.

406. Sealey, W.C., Boineau, J.P., and Wallace, A.G.: The identification and division of the bundle of Kent for premature ventricular excitation and supraventricular tachycardia, Surgery, 68:1009, 1970.

407. Donoso, E., Braunwald, E., Jick, S., and Grishman, A.: Congenital heart block, Am. J. Med., 20:869, 1956.

408. Engle, M.A., Ehlers, K.H., and Frand, M.: Natural history of congenital complete heart block, a cooperative study, Circulation, 42-111:112, 1970.

409. Scanlon, P.J., Pryor, R., and Bount, Jr., S.G.: Right bundle branch block associated with left superior or inferior intraventricular block: clinical setting, prognosis, and relation to complete heart block, Circulation, 42:1123, 1970.

410. _____ Pryor, R., and Blount, Jr., S.G.: Right bundle branch block associated with left superior or inferior intraventricular block: associated with acute myocardial infarction, Circulation, 42:1135, 1970.

411. Spach, M.S., Huang, S., Armstrong, S.I., and Canent, Jr., R.V.: Demonstration of peripheral conduction system in human hearts, Circulation, 38:333, 1963.

412. James, T.N., and Sherf, L.: Fine structure of the His bundle, Circulation, 44:9, 1971.

413. Cox, J.L., Daniel, T.M., Sabiston, D.C., and Boineau, J.P.: The electrophysiologic time-course of acute myocardial infarction and the effects of early coronary re-perfusion, Circulation, 42-111:98, 1970.

414. Cokkinos, D.V., Hallman, G.L., Cooley, D.A., Zamalloa, O., and Leachman, R.D.: Left ventricular aneurysm: analysis of electrocardiographic features and postresection changes, Am. Heart J., 82:149, 1971.

415. Rochmis, P., and Blackburn, H.: Exercise tests. A survey of procedures, safety, and litigation experience in approximately 170,-000 tests, J.A.M.A., 217:1061, 1971.

416. Okamoto, N., Kaneko, K., Simonson, E., and Schmitt, O.H.: Reliability of individual frontal plane axis determination, Circulation, 44:213, 1971.

417. Greenspan, K., Anderson, G.J., and Fisch, C.: Electrophysiologic correlate of exit block, Am. J. Cardiol., 28:197, 1971.

418. Myburgh, D.P., and Lewis, B.S.: Ventricular parasystole in healthy hearts, Am. Heart J., 82:307, 1971.

419. Ostrander, Jr., L.D.: Left axis deviation: prevalence, associated conditions, and prognosis. An epidemiologic study, Ann. Intern. Med., 75:23, 1971.

420. Rasmussen, K.: Chronic sino-atrial block, Am. Heart J., 81:38, 1971.

421. Easley, R.M., and Goldstein, S.: Sino-atrial syncope, Am. J. Med., 50:166, 1971.

422. Gunnar, R.M.: Cardiac conduction in patients with symptomatic sinus node disease, Circulation, 43:836, 1971.

423. Zipes, D.P.: Premature atrial contraction, Arch. Intern. Med., 128:453, 1971.

424. Chung, E.K.: A reappraisal of atrial dissociation, Am. J. Cardiol., 28:111, 1971.

425. Damato, A.N., and Lau, S.H.: Concealed and supernormal AV conduction, Circulation, 43:961, 1971.

426. Chung, E.K.: A reappraisal of concealed atrioventricular conduction, Am. Heart J., 82:408, 1971.

427. Parker, D.P., and Kaplan, M.A.: Demonstration of the supernormal period in the intact human heart as a result of pacemaker failure, Chest, 59:461, 1971.

428. Zipes, D.P., and Fisch, C.: Premature ventricular beats, Arch. Intern. Med., 128:140, 1971.

429. Rubenfire, M., Breneman, G.M., and Taber, R.E.: Entrance block: a previously unrecognized phenomenon associated with transthoracic demand pacemaker implantation, Am. Heart J., 81:102, 1971.

430. Goldreyer, B.N., Bigger, Jr., J.T.: Site of re-entry in paroxysmal supraventricular tachycardia in man, Circulation, 43:15, 1971.

431. Watanabe, Y.: Reassessment of parasystole, Am. Heart J., 81:451, 1971.

432. Proper, M.C., Ditchek, N.T., Purcell, A.D., and Smith, Jr., M.: Nonparoxysmal bidirectional rhythm, Chest, 59:333, 1971.

433. Perlman, L.V., Ostrander, Jr., L.D., Keller, J.B., and Chiang, B.N.: An epidemiologic study of first degree atrioventricular block in Tecumseh, Michigan, Chest, 59:400, 1971.

434. Haft, J.I., Weinstock, M., and DeGuia, R.: Electrophysiologic studies in Mobitz type II second degree heart block, Am. J. Cardiol., 27:682, 1971.

435. Wartak, J.: Computers in Electrocardiography, Springfield, Illinois, Charles C Thomas, 1970.

436. Caceres, C.A., and Dreifus, L.S. (Eds.): Clinical Electrocardiography and Computers, New York, Academic Press, Inc., 1970.

437. Stein, P.D., and Bruce, T.A.: Left axis deviation as an electrocardiographic manifestation of acute pulmonary embolism, J. Electrocardiol., 4:67, 1971.

438. Johnson, J.C., Flowers, N.D., and Horan, L.G.: Unexplained atrial flutter: a frequent herald of pulmonary embolism, Chest, 60:29, 1971.

439. Ohnell, R.F.: Pre-excitation: a cardiac abnormality. Pathophysiological, pathoanatomical, and clinical studies of an excitatory spread phenomenon, Acta Med. Scand., (Suppl) 152, 1944.

440. McHenry, P.L., Phillips, J.F., Fisch, C., and Corya, B.R.: Right precordial QRS pattern due to left anterior hemiblock, Am. Heart J., 81:498, 1971.

441. Horan, L.G., Flowers, N.C., and Johnson, J.C.: Significance of diagnostic Q wave of myocardial infarction, Circulation, 43:428, 1971.

442. Peterson, G.V., and Tikoff, G.: Left bundle branch block and left ventricular hypertrophy: electrocardiographic-pathologic correlations, Chest, 59:174, 1971.

443. Ewy, G.A., Karliner, J., and Bedynek, Jr., J.L.: Electrocardiographic QRS axis shift as a manifestation of hyperkalemia, J.A.M.A., 215:429, 1971.

444. Mariott, H.J.L., Schwartz, N.L., and Bix, H.H.: Ventricular fusion beats, Circulation, 26:880, 1962.

445. Kellerman, J.J.: Problems of exercise testing, Chest, 59:124, 1971.

446. Cohn, P.F., Vokonas, P.S., Herman, M.V., and Gorlin, R.: Postexercise electrocardiogram in patients with abnormal resting electrocardiograms, Circulation, 43:648, 1971.

447. Biberman, L., Sarma, R.N., and Surawicz, B.: T wave abnormalities during hyperventilation and isoproterenol infusion, Am. Heart J., 81:166, 1971.

448. Hanne-Paparo, N., Wendkos, M.H., and Brunner, D.: T wave abnormalities in the electrocardiograms of top-ranking athletes without demonstrable organic heart disease, Am. Heart J., 81:743, 1971.

449. Abildskov, J.A., Burgess, M.J., Millar, K., Wyatt, R., and Baule, G.: The primary T wave — a new electrocardiographic wave form, Am. Heart J., 81:242, 1971.

450. Haft, J.I., Herman, M.V., and Gorlin, R.: Left bundle branch block: etiologic, hemodynamic, and ventriculographic considerations, Circulation, 43:279, 1971.

451. Rosenbaum, M.B.: The hemiblocks: diagnostic criteria and clinical significance, Mod. Con. Cardiovasc. Dis., 39:141, 1970.

452. Braudo, M., Wigle, E.D., and Keith, J.D.: A distinctive electrocardiogram in muscular subaortic stenosis due to ventricular septal hypertrophy, Am. J. Cardiol., 14:599, 1964.

453. Han, J.: The concepts of reentrant activity responsible for ectopic rhythms, Am. J. Cardiol., 28:253, 1971.

454. Dreifus, L.S., and Watanabe, Y.: Localization and significance of atrioventricular block, Am. Heart J., 82:435, 1971.

455. Piccolo, E., Nava, A., and Della Volta, S.: Inferior atrial rhythms. Vectorcardiographic study and electrophysiologic considerations, Am. Heart J., 82:468, 1971.

456. Parisi, A.F., Beckmann, C.H., and Lancaster, M.C.: The spectrum of ST segment elevation in the electrocardiograms of healthy adult men, J. Electrocardiol., 4:137, 1971.

457. Zipes, D.P.: Premature AV junctional contractions, Arch. Intern. Med., 128:633, 1971.

458. Wolff, L., and Richman, J.L.: The diagnosis of myocardial infarction in patients with anomalous atrioventricular excitation (Wolff-Parkinson-White syndrome), Am. Heart J., 45:545, 1953.

459. Singer, D.H., and Eick, R.T.: Aberrancy: electrophysiologic aspects, Am. J. Cardiol., 28:381, 1971.

460. Fisch, C., Greenspan, K., and Anderson, G.J.: Exit block, Am. J. Cardiol., 28:402, 1971.

461. Moore, E.N., Knoebel, S., and Spear, J.F.: Concealed conduction, Am. J. Cardiol., 28:406, 1971.

462. James, T.N., and Sherf, L.: Specialized tissues and preferential conductions in the atria of the heart, Am. J. Cardiol., 28:414, 1971.

463. Narula, O.S., and Samet, P.: Right bundle branch block with normal, left, or right axis deviation. Analysis of His bundle recordings, Am. J. Med., 51:432, 1971.

464. Zipes, D.P., and Fisch, C.: Ventricular tachycardia, Arch. Intern. Med., 128:815, 1971.

465. Alexander, R.P.W., and Walker, B.F.: The bearing of race, sex, age, and nutritional state on the precordial electrocardiograms of young South African Bantu and Caucasian subjects, Am. Heart J., 77:441-459, 1969.

466. Seichi, A., Linde, L.M., Oshima, M., Momma, K., Nakamura, N., Yanagisawa, M., and Yoshine, K.: Isolated T-wave inversion in the electrocardiogram of children, Am. Heart J., 81:166-174, 1971.

467. Ashcroft, M.T., Miller, G.J., Beadnell, H.M.S.G., and Swan, A.V.: A comparison of T-wave inversion, ST elevation, and RS amplitudes in precordial leads of Africans and Indians in Guyana, Am. Heart J., 81:467-475, 1971.

468. Ishikawa, K., Berson, A.S., and Pipberger, H.V.: Electrocardio-

graphic changes due to cardiac enlargement, Am. Heart J., 81:635-643, 1971.

469. Dougherty, J.D.: The relation of QRS magnitude to the frontal QRS axis and the heart-electrode distance, J. of Electrocardiol., 4:249-260, 1971.

470. Brij, G.G., Hanson, C.S., and Han, J.: A-V conduction in hyper- and hypothyroid dogs, Am. Heart J., 83:504-511, 1972.

471. Wellens, H.J.J.: Isolated electrical alternans of the T wave, Chest, 62:319-321, 1972.

472. Bing, O.H.L., McDowell, J.W., Hartman, J., and Messer, J.V.: Pacemaker placement by ECG monitoring, N. Engl. J. Med., 287:651, 1972.

473. Dower, G.E., and Osborne, J.A.: Polarcardiographic study of hospital staff — abnormalities found in smokers, J. of Electrocardiol., 5:273-280, 1972.

474. Schifrin, B.S.: Fetal heart rate monitoring during labor, J.A.M.A., 222:184-189, 1972.

475. Greenburg, H., and Antin, S.: 1:1 conduction in atrial flutter after intravenous injection of aminophylline, J. of Electrocardiol., 5:391-394, 1972.

476. Sivertssen, E., and Jorganson, L.: Atrial dissocation, Am. Heart J., 85:103-107, 1973.

477. Frank, E.: An accurate, clinically practical system for spatial vectorcardiography, Circulation, 13:737, 1956.

478. Luy, G., Bahl, O.P., and Massie, E.: Intermittent left bundle branch block. A study of the effects of left bundle branch block on the electrocardiographic patterns of myocardial infarction and ischemia, Am. Heart J., 85:332, 1973.

479. Perosio, A.M., Suarez, L.D., and Llera, J.L.: Atrial dissociation, Am. Heart J., 85:401, 1973.

480. Kastor, J.A.: Digitalis intoxication in patients with atrial fibrillation, Circulation, 47:888, 1973.

481. Cohen, S.I., and Voukydis, P.: Disappearance of bundle branch block with slowing of normal heart rate, Am. Heart J., 85:727, 1973.

482. Gould, L., Venkataraman, K., Goswami, M.K., and Gomprecht, R.F.: Pacemaker-induced electrocardiographic changes simulating myocardial infarction, Chest, 63:829, 1973.

483. Lewis, S.M.: "Lead thirteen" electrocardiograph, J.A.M.A., 224:1533, 1973.

484. Schaal, S.F., Seidensticker, J., Goodman, R., and Wooley, C.F.: Familial right bundle branch block, left axis deviation, complete heart block, and early death, Ann. Intern. Med., 79:63, 1973.

485. Khan, A.H., Haider, R., Boughner, D.R., Oakley, C.M., and Good-

win, J.F.: Sinus rhythm with absent P waves in advanced rheumatic heart disease, Am. J. Cardiol., 32:93, 1973.

486. Pennington, K.S.: Advances in holography, Sci. Am. 218:40, 1968.
487. Scherlag, B.J., Lazzara, R., and Helfant, R.: Differentiation of "A-V junctional rhythms," Circulation, 48:304, 1973.
488. Tzivoni, D., and Stern, S.: Electrocardiographic pattern during sleep in healthy subjects and in patients with ischemic heart disease, J. of Electrocardiol., 6:225, 1973.
489. Shettigar, U.R., and Hultgren, J.: Lead thirteen electrocardiography, J.A.M.A., 226:78, 1973.
490. Fisch, C., Zipes, D.P., and McHenry, P.L.: Rate dependent aberrancy, Circulation, 48:714, 1973.
491. Dinari, G., and Aygen, M.M.: Sinoventricular conduction, N. Engl. J. Med., 289:1238, 1973.
492. Legato, M.J., and Ferrer, M.I.: Intermittent intra-atrial block: its diagnosis, incidence, and implications, Chest, 65:243, 1974.
493. Walston, A., Brewer, D.L., Kitchens, C.S., and Krook, J.E.: The electrocardiographic manifestations of spontaneous left pneumothorax, Ann. Intern. Med., 80:375, 1974.
494. Obel, I.W.P., Cohen, E., Millar, R.N.S.: Chronic symptomatic sinoatrial block: a review of 34 patients and their treatment, Chest, 65:397, 1974.
495. Bruce, R.A.: Methods of exercise testing. Step test, bicycle, treadmill, isometrics, Am. J. Cardiol., 33:715, 1974.
496. Shettigar, U.R., Hultgren, H.N., Pfeifer, J., and Lipton, M.J.: Diagnostic value of Q waves in inferior myocardial infarction, Am. Heart J., 88:170, 1974.
497. Bruce, R.A.: Exercise electrocardiography: pitfalls and solutions to interpretation, Circulation, 50:1, 1974.
498. Friedman, H.S., Gomes, J.A., Tardio, A., Levites, R., and Haft, J.I.: Appearance of atrial rhythm with absent P wave in longstanding atrial fibrillation, Chest, 66:172, 1974.
499. Cooksey, J.D., Parker, B.M., and Bahl, O.D.: The diagnostic contribution of exercise testing in left bundle branch block, Am. Heart J., 88:482, 1974.
500. Jacobs, W.F., Battle, W.E., and Ronan, J.A.: False-positive ST-T wave changes secondary to hyperventilation and exercise. A cineangiographic correlation, Arch. Intern. Med., 81:479, 1974.
501. Gradboys, T.B., and Majzoub, J.A.: Smudge, ECG., N. Engl. J. Med., 292:50, 1975.
502. Tuqan, S., Mau, R.D., and Schwartz, M.J.: Anterior myocardial infarction patterns in the mitral valve prolapse-systolic click syndrome, Am. J. of Med., 58:719, 1975.
503. Hammer, W.J., Luessenhop, A.J., and Weintraub, A.M.: Obser-

vations on electrocardiographic changes associated with subarachnoid hemorrhage with special reference to their genesis, Am. J. of Med., 59:427, 1975.

504. Nizet, P.M., Borgia, J.F., and Horvath, S.M.: Wandering atrial pacemaker (prevalence in French hornists), J. of Electrocardiol., 9:51 (1), 1976.

505. Stuart, Jr., R.H., and Ellestad, M.H.: Upsloping ST segments in exercise stress testing. Six year follow-up study of 438 patients and correlation with 248 angiograms, Am. J. Cardiol., 37:19, 1976.

506. Engel, T.R., Bond, R.C., and Schall, S.F.: First degree sino-atrial heart block: sino-atrial block in the sick-sinus syndrome, Am. Heart J., 91:303, 1976.

507. Massing, G.K., and James, T.N.: Anatomical configuration of the His bundle and bundle branch in the human heart, Circulation, 53:609, 1976.

508. Das, G.: Left axis deviation: a spectrum of intraventricular conduction block, Circulation, 53:917, 1976.

509. Chaudron, J.M., Heller, F., Van den Berghe, H.B., and LeBacq, E.G.: Attacks of ventricular fibrillation and unconsciousness in a patient with prolonged QT interval. A family study, Am. Heart J., 91:783, 1976.

510. Kambara, H., and Phillips, J.: Long-term evaluation of early repolarization syndrome (normal varient RS-T segment evaluation), Am. J. Cardiol., 38:157, 1976.

511. Farnham, D.J., and Shah, P.M.: Left anterior hemiblock simulating anteroseptal myocardial infarction, Am. Heart J., 92:363, 1976.

512. Spodick, D.H.: Pericarditis vs. early repolarization: electrocardiographic differentiation, N. Engl. J. Med., 295:523, 1976.

513. Bertrand, C.A.: Computer analysis of the electrocardiogram, Am. J. Cardiol., 38:394, 1976.

514. Caceres, C.A.: Limitations of computer in electrocardiographic interpretation, Am. J. Cardiol., 38:362, 1976.

515. Sheffield, L.T., and Reitman, D.: Stress testing methodology, Prog. Cardiovasc. Dis., 19:33, 1976.

516. Arnsdorff, M.F.: Electrocardiogram in hyperkalemia, Arch. Intern. Med., 136:1161, 1976.

517. Kuritzky, P., and Goldfarb, A.L.: Unusual electrocardiographic changes in spontaneous pneumothorax, Chest, 70:535, 1976.

518. Kulbertus, H.E.: Reevaluation of the prognosis of patients with LAD-RBBB, Am. Heart J., 92:665, 1976.

519. Zipes, D.P., Gaum, W.E., Genetos, B.C., Glassman, R.D., Noble, R.J., and Fisch, C.: Atrial tachycardia without P waves masquerading as an AV junctional tachycardia, Circulation, 55:253, 1977.

520. Wang, K., Goldfarb, B.L., Gobel, F.L., and Armstrong, D.: Multi-focal atrial tachycardia, Arch. Intern. Med., 137:161, 1977.

521. Jordan, J.L., Yamaguchi, I., and Mandel, W.J.: The sick sinus syndrome, J.A.M.A., 237:682, 1977.

522. Wiberg, T.A., Richman, H.G., and Gobel, F.L.: The significance and prognosis of chronic bifascicular block, Chest, 71:329, 1977.

523. Whinnery, J.E., Froelicher, Jr., V.F., Stewart, A.J., Longo, Jr., M.R., and Triebwasser, J.H.: The electrocardiographic response to maximal treadmill exercise of asymptomatic men with right bundle branch block, Chest, 71:335, 1977.

524. Singer, D.H., Wicks, J., Ten Eick, R.E., and DeBoer, A.: Atrial dissociation: possible cellular electrophysiologic mechanisms, Am. J. of Med., 62:643, 1977.

525. Rotmensch, H.H., Meytes, I., Terdiman, R., and Laniado, S.: Incidence and significance of the low-voltage electrocardiogram in acute myocardial infarction, Chest, 71:708, 1977.

526. Gupta, P.K., Lichstein, E., and Chadda, K.D.: Follow-up studies in patients with right bundle branch block and left anterior hemiblock: significance of H-V interval, J. of Electrocardiol., 10:221, 1977.

527. Zohman, L.A., and Kattus, A.A.: Exercise testing in the diagnosis of coronary heart disease, Am. J. Cardiol., 40:243, 1977.

528. Ibrahim, M.M., Tarazi, R.C., Dustan, H.P., and Gifford, Jr., R.W.: Electrocardiogram in evaluation of resistance to antihypertensive therapy, Arch. Intern. Med., 137:1125, 1977.

529. Guyton, R.A., McClenathan, J.H., Newman, G.E., and Michaelis, L.E.: Significance of subendocardial ST segment elevation caused by coronary stenosis in the dog. Epicardial ST segment depression, local ischemia, and subsequent necrosis, Am. J. Cardiol., 40:373, 1977.

530. Rifkin, R.D., and Hood, W.B.: Bayesian analysis of electrocardiographic exercise stress testing, N. Engl. J. Med., 297:681, 1977.

531. Olveros, R.A., Seaworth, J., Weiland, F.L., and Boucher, C.A.: Intermittent left anterior hemiblock during treadmill exercise test, Chest, 72:492, 1977.

532. Mimbs, J.W., de Mello, V., and Roberts, R.: The effect of respiration on normal and abnormal Q waves. An electrocardiographic and vectorcardiographic analysis, Am. Heart J., 94:579, 1977.

533. Ferrer, M.I.: The sick sinus syndrome: its status after ten years, Chest, 72:554, 1977.

534. Hoffman, I.: Anterior conduction delay, Am. Heart J., 94:813, 1977.

535. Ogawa, S., Dreifus, L.S., and Osmick, M.J.: Longitudinal dissociation of Bachman's bundle as a mechanism of supraventricular tachycardia, Am. J. Cardiol., 40:915, 1977.

536. James, T.N.: The sinus node, Am. J. Cardiol., 40:965, 1977.

537. Tokon, M.J., Lee, G., DeMaria, A.N., Miller, R.R., and Mason, D.T.: Effects of digitalis on the exercise electrocardiogram in normal adult subjects, Chest, 72:714, 1977.

538. Magram, M., and Lee, Y.-C.: The pseudo-infarction pattern of left anterior hemiblock, Chest, 72:771, 1977.

539. Nemati, M., Doyle, J.T., McCaughan, D., Dunn, R.A., and Pipberger, H.V.: The orthogonal electrocardiogram in normal women. Implications of sex differences in diagnostic electrocardiography, Am. Heart J., 95:12, 1978.

540. Iwamura, N., Kodama, I., Shimizu, T., Hirata, Y., Toyama, J., and Yamada, K.: Functional properties of the left septal Purkinje network in premature activation of the ventricular conduction system, Am. Heart J., 95:60, 1978.

541. Stephan, E.: Hereditary bundle branch system defect. Survey of a family with four affected generations, Am. Heart J., 95:89, 1978.

542. Faris, J.V., McHenry, P.L., and Morris, S.N.: Concepts and applications of treadmill exercise testing and the exercise electrocardiogram, Am. Heart J., 95:102, 1978.

543. Nakaya, Y., Hiasa, Y., Murayama, Y., Ueda, S., Nagao, T., Niki, T., Mori, H., and Takashima, Y.: Prominent anterior QRS forces as a manifestation of left septal fascicular block, J. of Electrocardiol., 11:39, 1978.

544. Engel, T.R., Meister, S.G., and Frankl, W.S.: The "R-on-T" phenomenon, Ann. Intern. Med., 88:221, 1978.

545. Navarro-Lopez, F., Cinca, J., Sanz, G., Periz, A., Magrina, J., and Betriu, A.: Isolated T wave alternans, Am. Heart J., 95:369, 1978.

546. Narula, O.S.: The manifestation of bundle branch block due to lesions within the His bundle: a dilemma in electrocardiographic interpretations, Chest, 73:312, 1978.

547. Dowel, R.T., and McManus, III, R.E.: Pressure-induced cardiac enlargement in neonatal and adult rats: left ventricular functional characteristics and evidence of cardiac muscle proliferation in the neonate, Circ. Res., 42:303, 1978.

548. Pastore, J.O., Yurchak, P.M., Janis, K.M., Murphy, J.D., and Zir, L.M.: The risk of advanced heart block in surgical patients with right bundle branch block and left axis deviation, Circulation, 57:677, 1978.

549. Tanaka, T., Friedman, M.J., Okada, R.D., Buckels, L.J., and Marcus, F.I.: Diagnostic value of exercise-induced ST segment depression in patients with right bundle branch block, Am. J. Cardiol., 41:670, 1978.

550. Ariet, M., and Crevasse, L.E.: Status report on computerized ECG analysis, J.A.M.A., 239:1201, 1978.

551. Bonoris, P.E., Greenberg, P.S., Christison, G.W., Castellanet, M.J., and Ellestad, M.H.: Evaluation of R wave amplitude changes versus ST-segment depression in stress testing, Circulation, 57:904, 1978.

552. Keller, D.H., and Johnson, J.B.: The T wave of the unipolar precordial electrocardiogram in normal adult Negro subjects, Am. Heart J., 44:494, 1952.

553. Wasserberger, R.H., Alt, W.J., and Lloyd, C.J.: The normal RS-T elevation variant, Am. J. Cardiol., 8:184, 1961.

554. Lichtman, J., O'Rourke, R., Klein, A., and Karliner, J.S.: Electrocardiogram of the athlete. Alterations simulating those of organic heart disease, Arch. Intern. Med., 132:763, 1973.

555. Raunio, H., Rissanen, V., Jokinen, C., and Penttila, O.: Significance of a terminal R wave in lead V1 of the electrocardiogram, Am. Heart J., 95:702, 1978.

556. HHO/ISC Task Force: Definition of terms related to cardiac rhythm, Am. Heart J., 95:796, 1978.

557. Scherlag, B.J., Lazzara, R., and Helfant, R.H.: Differentiation of "Av junctional rhythms," Circulation, 48:304, 1973.

558. Friesinger, G.C., and Smith, R.F.: Correlation of electrocardiographic studies and arteriographic findings with angina pectoris, Circulation, 46:1173, 1972.

559. McNamara, J.J., Molt, M.A., Streple, J.F., and Cutting, R.T.: Coronary artery disease in combat casualties in Vietnam, J.A.M.A., 216:1185, 1971.

560. Schubart, A.F., Marriott, H.J.L., and Gorten, R.J.: Isorhythmic dissociation. Atrioventricular dissociation with synchronization, Am. J. of Med., 24:209, 1958.

561. Herrick, J.B.: An intimate account of my early experience with coronary thrombosis, Am. Heart J., 27:1, 1944.

562. Smith, F.M.: The ligation of coronary arteries with electrocardiographic study, Arch. Intern. Med., 22:8, 1918.

563. Mattingly, T.W.: The postexercise electrocardiogram: its value in the diagnosis and prognosis of coronary arterial disease, Am. J. Cardiol., 9:395, 1962.

564. Feil, H., and Siegel, M.L.: Electrocardiographic changes during attacks of angina pectoris, Am. J. Med. Sci., 175:255, 1928.

565. Orzan, F., Garcia, E., Mathur, V.S., and Hall, R.J.: Is the treadmill test useful for evaluating coronary artery disease in patients with complete left bundle branch block? Am. J. Cardiol., 42:36, 1978.

566. Doan, A.E., Peterson, D.R., Blackmon, J.R., and Bruce, R.A.: Myocardial ischemia after maximal exercise in healthy men. A method for detecting potential coronary heart disease? Am. Heart J., 69:11, 1965.

567. Blumgart, H.L.: Coronary disease: clinical-pathologic correlations

and physiology, Bull. N.Y. Acad. Med., 27:693, 1951.

568. Enos, W.F., Holmes, R.H., and Beyer, J.: Coronary artery disease among United States soldiers killed in action in Korea: preliminary report, J.A.M.A., 152:1090, 1953.

569. Chou, T.-C., and Wenzke, F.: The importance of R on T phenomenon, Am. Heart J., 96:191, 1978.

570. Henson, J.R.: Descartes and the ECG lettering system, J. His. Med., 26:181, 1971.

571. Hayakawa, S.I.: Language in Thought and Action, 3rd ed., Harcourt Brace Jovanovich, Inc., New York, 1972.

572. Weitzenbaum, J.: Computer Power and Human Reason: From Judgment to Calculation, W.H. Freemen and Company, San Francisco, 1976.

573. Mann, H.: A method of analyzing the electrocardiogram, Arch. Intern. Med., 25:283, 1920.

574. Comroe, Jr., J.H., Retrospectroscope. Insights Into Medical Discovery, Von Gehr Press, Menlo Park, California, 1977.

575. MacKenzie, Sir J.: Diseases of the Heart, 4th ed., Oxford University Press, London, 1925.

576. Goodman, L.S., and Gilman, A.: The Pharmacologics of Therapeutics, 2nd ed., Macmillan, New York, 1955.

577. Marriott, H.J.L.: Practical Electrocardiography, 6th ed., Williams & Wilkins, Baltimore, 1977.

578. Lamberti, J.J., Silver, H., Howell, J., Kampman, K., and Glagov, S.: Transmural gradients of experimental myocardial ischemia: limited correlation of ultrastructure with epicardial ST segment, Am. Heart J., 96:496, 1978.

579. Norman, T.D., and Coers, C.D.: Cardiac hypertrophy after coronary ligation in rats, Arch. Pathol., 69:181, 1960.

580. Reiffel, J.A., and Bigger, J.T.: Pure anterior conduction delay: a variant "fascicular" defect, J. of Electrocardiol., 11(4):315, 1978.

581. Nelson, C.V., Lange, R.L., Hecht, H.H., Carlisle, R.P., and Ruby, A.S.: Effect of intracardiac blood and of fluids of different conductivities on the magnitude of surface vectors, Circulation, 14:977, 1956 (Abstract).

582. Nelson, C.V., Chatterjee, M., Angelakos, E.T., and Hecht, H.H.: Model studies on the effect of the intracardiac blood on the electrocardiogram, Am. Heart J., 62:83, 1961.

583. Angelakos, E.T., and Gokhan, N.: Influence of venous inflow volume on the QRS potential "in vivo," Cardiologia, 42:377, 1963.

584. Dern, P.K., Pryor, R., Walker, S.H., and Searls, D.T.: Serial electrocardiographic changes in treated hypertensive patients with reference to voltage criteria, mean QRS vectors, and the QRS-T angle,

Circulation, 36:823, 1967.

585. Doyle, A.E., Electrocardiographic changes in hypertension treated by methonium compounds, Am. Heart J., 45:363, 1953.

586. Sigler, L.H.: Abnormalities in the electrocardiogram induced by emotional strain, Am. J. Cardiol., 8:807, 1961.

587. Spodick, D.H.: Acute cardiac tamponade: pathologic physiology, diagnosis, and management, Prog. Cardiovasc. Dis., 10:84, 1967.

588. Blackburn, H., Vasquez, C.L., and Keys, A.: The aging electrocardiogram: a common aging process or latent coronary artery disease, Am. J. Cardiol., 20:618, 1967.

589. Toney, J.C., and Kolmen, S.N.: Cardiac tamponade: fluid and pressure effects on electrocardiographic changes, Proc. Soc. Exp. Biol. Med., 121:642, 1966.

590. Wilson, F.N.: The distribution of potential differences produced by the heartbeat within the body and at its surface, Am. Heart J., 5:599 (#3), 1930.

591. Hamlin, R.L., Pipers, F.S., Hellerstein, H.K., and Smith, R.: Alterations in QRS during ischemia of the left ventricular free-wall in goats, J. of Electrocardiol., 2(3):223, 1969.

592. Kilty, S.E., Lepeschkin, E.: Effect of body build on the QRS voltage of the electrocardiogram in normal men. Its significance in the diagnosis of left ventricular hypertrophy, Circulation, 31:77, 1965.

593. Grubschmidt, H.A., and Sokolow, M.: The reliability of high voltage of the QRS complex as a diagnostic sign of left ventricular hypertrophy in adults, Am. Heart J., 54:689, 1957.

594. Harris, S.A., and Randall, W.C.: Mechanisms underlying electrocardiographic changes observed in anoxia, Am. J. of Physiol., 142:452, 1944.

595. Greenspahn, B.R., Barzilai, B., and Denes, P.: Electrocardiographic changes in concussion, Chest, 74:447, 1978.

596. Gould, W.L.: Auricular fibrillation: report on a study of a familial tendency, 1920–1956, Arch. Intern. Med., 100:916, 1957.

597. Rosenfeld, I.: Personal communication, 1978.

598. Vismara, L.A., Vera, Z., Miller, R.R., and Mason, D.T.: Efficacy of disopyramide phosphate in the treatment of refractory ventricular tachycardia, Am. J. Cardiol., 39:1027, 1977.

599. Woosley, R.L., and Shand, D.G.: Pharmacokinetics of antiarrhythmic drugs, Am. J. Cardiol., 41:986, 1978.

600. Zipes, D.P., and Troup, P.J.: New antiarrhythmic agents, Am. J. Cardiol., 41:1005, 1978.

601. Danilo, Jr., P.: Cardiac effects of disopyramide, Am. Heart J., 92:532, 1976.

602. Helfant, R.H.: Coronary arterial spasm and provocative testing in

ischemic heart disease, Am. J. Cardiol., 41:787, 1978.

603. Heupler, Jr., F.A., Proudfit, W.L., Razavi, M., Shirley, E.K., Green-street, R., and Sheldon, W.C.: Ergonovine maleate provocative test for coronary arterial spasm, Am. J. Cardiol., 41:631, 1978.

604. Manoach, M., Gitter, S., Grossman, E., Varon, D., and Gassner, S.: Influence of hemorrhage on the QRS complex of the electrocardiogram, Am. Heart J., 82:55, 1971.

605. Toshima, H., Koga, Y., and Kimura, N.: Correlations between electrocardiographic, vectorcardiographic, and echocardiographic findings in patients with left ventricular overload, Am. Heart J., 94:547, 1977.

606. Bennett, D.: Main determinant of ECG voltage measurements, Am. Heart J., 96:835, 1978.

607. Kenelly, B.M., and Lane, G.K.: Electrophysiological studies in four patients with atrial flutter with 1:1 atrioventricular conduction, Am. Heart J., 96:723, 1978.

608. Broome, R.A., Estes, Jr., E.H., and Orgain, E.S.: The effects of digitoxin upon the twelve lead electrocardiogram, Am. J. of Med., 21:237, 1956.

609. Pick, A.: Digitalis and the electrocardiogram, Circulation, 15:603, 1957.

610. Harrison, D.C., Fitzgerald, J.W., and Winkle, R.A.: Ambulatory ECG's to diagnose and treat cardiac arrhythmias, N. Engl. J. Med., 294:373, 1976.

611. Krasnow, A.Z., and Bloomfield, D.K.: Artifacts in portable electrocardiographic monitoring, Am. Heart J., 91:349, 1976.

612. Janse, M.J., Anderson, R.H., van Capelle, F.J.L., and Durrer, D.: A combined electrophysiological and anatomical study of the human fetal heart, Am. Heart J., 91:556, 1976.

613. Penchas, S., and Keynan, A.: False myocardial infarction pattern in the ECG of a patient with funnel-chest, J. of Electrocardiol., 2:285, 1969.

614. Watanabe, Y., Nishijima, K., Richman, H., and Simonson, E.: Vectorcardiographic and electrocardiographic differentiation between cor pulmonale and anterior wall myocardial infarction, Am. Heart J., 84:302, 1972.

615. Summers, R.S.: The electrocardiogram as a diagnostic aid in pneumothorax, Chest, 63:127, 1973.

616. Jackson, D.H., and Murphy, G.W.: Nonpenetrating cardiac trauma, Mod. Con. Cardiovasc. Dis., 45:123, 1976.

617. Miller, R., Ward, C., Amsterdam, E., Mason, D.T., and Zelis, R.: Focal mononucleosis myocarditis simulating myocardial infarction, Chest, 63:102, 1973.

618. Ruskin, J.N., Akthar, M., Damato, A.N., Ticzon, A.R., Lau, S.H., and Caracta, A.R.: Abnormal Q waves in Wolff-Parkinson-White syndrome. Incidence and clinical significance, J.A.M.A., 235:2727, 1976.

619. Roberts, W.C., McAllister, Jr., H.A., and Ferrans, V.J.: Sarcoidosis of the heart. A clinicopathologic study of 35 necropsy patients (Group I) and review of previously described necropsy patients (Group II), Am. J. of Med., 63:86, 1977.

620. Zatuchni, J., and Baute, A.: Duchenne electrocardiogram in myotonia congenita, J. of Electrocardiol., 11(4):395, 1978.

621. Lemberg, L.: Coexisting left anterior hemiblock and inferior wall infarction, Chest, 69:333, 1976.

622. Moleiro, F., Mendoza, I.: Left anterior hemiblock of the 2:1 type in the presence of inferior wall myocardial infarction, Chest, 69:418, 1976.

623. Hoffman, I., Mehta, J., Hilsenrath, J., and Hamby, R.I.: Anterior conduction delay: a possible cause for prominent anterior QRS forces, J. of Electrocardiol., 9:15, (1), 1976.

624. Salem, B.I., Schnee, M., Leatherman, L., de Castro, C.M., and Benrey, J.: Electrocardiographic pseudo-infraction pattern: appearance with a large posterior pericardial effusion after cardiac surgery, Am. J. Cardiol., 42:681, 1978.

625. Margolis, J.R., Kannel, W.B., Feinleib, M., Dawber, T.R., and McNamara, P.M.: Clinical features of unrecognized myocardial infarction — silent and symptomatic. Eighteen years follow-up: the Framingham study, Am. J. Cardiol., 32:1, 1973.

626. Zeft, H.J., Friedberg, H.D., King, J.F., Manley, J.C., Houston, J.H., and Johnson, W.D.: Reappearance of anterior QRS forces after coronary bypass surgery. An electrovectorcardiographic study, Am. J. Cardiol., 36:163, 1975.

627. Conde, C.A., Meller, J., Espinoza, J., Donoso, E., and Dack, S.: Disappearance of abnormal Q waves after aortocoronary bypass surgery, Am. J. Cardiol., 36:889, 1975.

628. Altieri, P., and Schaal, S.F.: Inferior and anteroseptal myocardial infarction concealed by transient left anterior hemiblock, Am. J. Cardiol., 6:257, 1973.

629. Dodek, A., and Neill, W.A.: Corrected transposition of the great arteries, masquerading as a coronary artery disease, Am. J. Cardiol., 30:910, 1972.

630. Sheffield, L.T., Holt, J.H., and Reeves, T.J.: Exercise graded by heart rate in electrocardiographic testing for angina pectoris, Circulation, 32:622, 1965.

631. Surawicz, B., and Saito, S.: Exercise testing for detection of myocar-

dial ischemia in patients with abnormal electrocardiograms at rest, Am. J. Cardiol., 41:943, 1978.

632. Minow, R.A., Benjamin, R.S., Lee, E.T., and Gottlieb, J.A.: QRS voltage change with adriamycin administration, Cancer Treat. Rep., 62:931, 1978.

633. Rhinehart, J.J., Lewis, R.B., and Balcerzak, S.P.: Adriamycin cardiotoxicity in man, Ann. Intern. Med., 81:475, 1974.

634. Usher, B.W., and Popp, R.L.: Electrical alternans: mechanism in pericardial effusion, Am. Heart J., 83:459, 1972.

635. Colvin, J.: Electrical alternans: case report and comments on the literature, Am. Heart J., 55:513, 1958.

636. Spodick, D.H.: Electrical alternans, Am. Heart J., 84:574, 1972.

637. Spodick, D.H.: Electrical alternation of the heart. Its relation to the kinetics and physiology of the heart during cardiac tamponade, Am. J. Cardiol., 10:155, 1962.

638. Littman, D.: Alternation of the heart, Circulation, 27:280, 1963.

639. Wasserburger, R.H., Kelly, J.R., Rasmussen, H.K., and Juhl, J.H.: The electrocardiographic pentalogy of pulmonary emphysema. A correlation of roentgenographic findings and pulmonary function studies, Circulation, 20:831, 1959.

640. Carilli, A.D., Denson, L.J., and Timmapuri, N.: Electrocardiographic estimation of pulmonary impairment in chronic obstruction lung disease, Chest, 63:483, 1973.

641. Kamper, D., Chou, T.-C., Fowler, N.O., Witt, R.L., and Bloomfield, S.: The reliability of electrocardiographic criteria for chronic obstructive lung disease, Am. Heart J., 80:445, 1970.

642. Littman, D.: The electrocardiographic findings in pulmonary emphysema, Am. J. Cardiol., 5:339, 1960.

643. Cheng, T.O., and Bashour, T.T.: Striking electrocardiographic changes associated with pheochromocytoma, Chest, 70:397, 1976.

644. Wang, K., Segal, M., and Ward, P.C.J.: Sudden disappearance of electrocardiographic pattern of anteroseptal myocardial infarction: result of superimposed acute posterior infarction, Chest, 70:402, 1976.

645. Burch, G.E.: Of the PR segment depression and atrial infarction, Am. Heart J., 91:129, 1976.

646. Kleiner, J.P., Nelson, W.P., Boland, M.J.: The 12-lead electrocardiogram in exercise testing. A misleading baseline? Arch. Intern. Med., 138:1572, 1978.

647. McAnulty, J.H., Rahimtoola, S., Murphy, E.S., Kauffman, S., Ritzmann, L.W., Kanarek, P., and DeMots, H.: A prospective study of sudden death in "high risk" bundle branch block, N. Engl. J. Med., 299:209, 1978.

648. Benditt, D.G., Pritchett, E.L.C., Smith, W.M., Wallace, A.G., and Gallagher, J.J.: Characteristics of atrioventricular conduction and the spectrum of arrhythmias in Lown-Ganong-Levine syndrome, Circulation, 57:454, 1978.

649. Joseph, M.E., and Kastor, J.A.: Superventricular tachycardia in Lown-Ganong-Levine syndrome: atrionodal versus intranodal re-entry, Am. J. Cardiol., 40:521, 1977.

650. Ferrer, M.I.: Preexcitaiton, Am. J. of Med., 62:715, 1977.

651. Grayzel, J., and Angeles, J.: Sino-atrial block in man provoked by quinidine, J. of Electrocardiol., 5:289, 1972.

652. Talano, J.V., Euler, D., Randall, W.C., Eshaghy, B., Loeb, H.S., and Gunnar, R.M.: Sinus node dysfunction. An overview with emphasis on autonomic and pharmacologic consideration, Am. J. of Med., 64:773, 1978.

653. Yabek, S.M., Swensson, R.E., and Jarmakani, J.M.: Electrocardiographic recognition of sinus node dysfunction in children and adults, Circulation, 56:235, 1977.

654. Thery, C., Gosselin, B., Lekieffre, J., and Warembourg, H.: Pathology of sinoatrial node. Correlations with electrocardiographic findings in 111 patients, Am. Heart J., 93:735, 1977.

655. Kaplinsky, E., Aronson, R., and Neufeld, H.N.: Isorhythmic dissociation — a "physiological" arrhythmia, J. of Electrocardiol., 10:179, 1977.

656. Moe, G.K., Jalife, J., Mueller, W.J., and Moe, B.: A mathematical model of parasystole and its application to clinical arrhythmias, Circulation, 56:968, 1977.

657. Moss, H.J., and Schwartz, P.J.: Sudden death and the idiopathic long Q-T syndrome, Am. J. of Med., 66:6, 1979.

658. Gay, R., and Brown, D.F.: Bradycardia-dependent bundle branch block in acute myocardial infarction, Chest, 64:114, 1973.

659. Simpson, Jr., R.J., Rosenthal, H.M., Rimmer, Jr., R.H., and Foster, J.R.: Alternating bundle branch block, Chest, 74:447, 1978.

660. Dhingra, R.C., Amat-Y-Leon, F., Windham, C., Sridhar, S.S., Wu, D., Denes, P., and Rosen, K.M.: Significance of left axis deviation in patients with chronic left bundle branch block, Am. J. Cardiol., 42:551, 1978.

661. Aiegman-Igra, Y., Yahini, J.H., Goldbourt, U., and Neufeld, H.: Intraventricular conduction disturbances: a review of prevalence, etiology, and progression for ten years within a stable population of Israeli adult males, Am. Heart J., 96:669, 1978.

662. Lev, M.: The pathology of complete AV block, Prog. Cardiovasc. Dis., 6:317, 1964.

663. Lenegre, J.: Etiology and pathology of bilateral bundle branch block

in relation to complete heart bloc, Prog. Cardiovasc. Dis., 6:409, 1964.

664. Eraker, S.A., Wickamasekeran, R., and Goldman, S.: Complete heart block with hyperthyroidism, J.A.M.A., 239:1644, 1978

665. Gambetta, M., and Childers, R.W.: Rate-dependent right precordial Q waves: "septal focal block," Am. J. Cardiol., 32:196, 1973.

666. Danzig, M.D., Robertson, T.L., Webber, L.S., Day, G., and Dock, D.S.: Earlier onset of QRS in anterior precordial ECG leads: precision of time interval measurements, Circulation, 54:447, 1976.

667. Igarashi, M., and Ayabe, T.: Quantitative study of the supernormal phase of ventricular excitability in man, Am. J. Cardiol., 36:292, 1975.

668. Hashimoto, K., Corday, E., Lang, T.-W., Meerbaum, S., Osher, J., Farcot, J.-C., and Davidson, R.M.: Significance of ST segment elevations in acute myocardial ischemia. Evaluation with intracoronary electrode techniques, Am. J. Cardiol., 37:493, 1976.

669. Wasserburger, R.H., Alt, W.J., and Lloyd, C.J.: The normal RS-T segment elevation variant, Am. J. Cardiol., 8:184, 1961.

670. Watanabe, Y.: Purkinje repolarization as a possible cause of the U wave in the electrocardiogram, Circulation, 51:1030, 1975.

671. Schwartz, P.J., and Malliani, A.: Electrical alternation of the T wave: clinical and experimental evidence of its relationship with the sympathetic nervous system and with the long Q-T syndrome, Am. Heart J., 89:45, 1975.

672. Allen, R.D., Gettes, L.S., Phalan, C., and Avington, M.D.: Painless ST segment depression in patients with angina pectoris: correlation with daily activities and cigarette smoking, Chest, 69:467, 1976.

673. Flowers, N.C., Horan, L.G., and Johnson, J.C.: Anterior infarctional changes occurring during mid and late ventricular activation detectable by surface mapping techniques, Circulation, 54:906, 1976.

674. Savage, R.M., Wagner, G.S., Ideker, R.E., Podolsky, S.A., and Hackel, D.B.: Correlation of postmortem anatomic findings with electrocardiographic changes in patients with myocardial infarction, Circulation, 55:279, 1977.

675. Scheinman, M.M., and Abbott, J.A.: Clinical significance of transmural versus nontransmural electrocardiographic changes in patients with acute myocardial infarction, Am. J. of Med., 55:602, 1973.

676. Abbott, J.A., and Scheinman, M.M.: Nondiagnostic electrocardiogram in patients with acute myocardial infarction. Clinical and anatomic correlations, Am. J. of Med., 55:608, 1973.

677. Ali, M., Cohen, H.C., and Singer, D.H.: ECG diagnosis of acute myocardial infarction in patients with pacemakers, Arch. Intern. Med., 138:1534, 1978.

678. Akhtar, M., and Damato, A.N.: Clinical uses of His bundle electrocardiography. Part I, Am. Heart J., 91:520, 1976.

679. Stern, S., and Tzivoni, D.: On artifacts in portable electrocardiographic monitoring, Am. Heart J., 94:131, 1977.

680. McGowan, R.L., Martin, N.D., Zaret, B.L., Hall, R.R., Bryson, A.L., Strauss, H.W., and Flamm, M.D.: Diagnostic accuracy of noninvasive myocardial imaging for coronary artery disease: an electrocardiographic and echocardiographic correlation, Am. J. Cardiol., 40:6, 1977.

681. Rapaport, A., Sepp, A.H., and Brown, W.H.: Carcinoma of the parathyroid gland with pulmonary metastases and cardiac death, Am. J. of Med., 28:443, 1960.

682. Gordon, A.J., Vagueiro, M.C., and Barold, S.S.: Endocardial electrograms from pacemaker catheters, Circulation, 38:82, 1968.

683. Green, H.L.: Clinical applications of His bundle electrocardiography, J.A.M.A., 240:258, 1978.

684. Madias, J.E., and Hood, W.B.: Value and limitations of precordial ST segment mapping, Arch. Intern. Med., 138:529, 1978.

685. Kennedy, H.L., and Caralis, D.G.: Ambulatory electrocardiography. A clinical perspective, Ann. Intern. Med., 87:729, 1977.

686. Bonner, R.E., and Schwetman, H.E.: Computer diagnosis of electrocardiograms II. A computer program for EKG measurements, Comput. Biomed. Res., 1:366, 1968.

687. Pipberger, H.V., and Cornfield, J.: What computer program to choose for clinical application: the need for consumer protection, Circulation, 47:918, 1973.

688. Einthovan, W.: Le telecardiogramme, Arch. Int. Physiol. 4:132, 1906.

689. Vincent, G.M., Abildskov, J.A., and Burgess, M.J.: QT interval syndromes, Prog. Cardiovasc. Dis., 16:523, 1974.

690. Schwartz, P.J., Periti, M., and Malliani, A.: The long Q-T syndrome, Am. Heart J., 89:378, 1975.

691. Alboni, P., Malacarne, C., DeLorenzi, E., Pirani, R., Baldassarri, F., and Masoni, A.: Right precordial Q waves due to superior fascicular block. Clinical and vectorcardiographic study, J. of Electrocardiol., 12:41, (1), 1979.

692. Ribeiro, L.G.T., Louie, E.K., Hillis, L.D., Davis, M.A., and Maroko, P.R.: Early augmentation of R wave voltage after coronary occlusion: a useful index of myocardial injury, J. of Electrocardiol., 12:89, (1), 1978.

693. Devereux, R.B., Perloff, J.K., Reichnek, N., and Josephson, M.E.: Mitral valve prolapse, Circulation, 54:3, 1976.

694. Dhingra, R.C., Wyndham, C., Amat-y-Leon, F., Denes, P., Wu, D.,

Sridhar, S., Bustin, A.G., and Rosen, K.M.: Incidence and site of AV block in patients with chronic bifascicular block, Circulation, 59:238, 1979.

695. Jervell, A., and Lange-Nielsen, F.: Congenital deaf-mutism, functional heart disease with prolongation of the Q-T interval, and sudden death, Am. Heart J., 54:59, 1957.

696. Segers, M., Lequime, J., and Denolin, H.: L'activitation ventriculaire precoce de certains couers hyperexeitables. Etude d l'onde delta de l'ectrocardiogramme, Cardiologia, 8:113, 1944.

697. Chen, C.-H., Nobuyoshi, M., and Kawai, C.: ECG pattern of left ventricular hypertrophy in nonobstructive hypertrophic cardiomyopathy: the significance of the mid-precordial changes, Am. Heart J., 97:687, 1979.

698. Shapiro, E.: Engelmann and his laddergram, Am. J. Cardiol., 39:464, 1977.

699. Athanassopoulos, C.B.: Transient focal septal block, Chest, 75:728, 1979.

Index

Abberation, ventricular, 68, 95
Acceleration of junctional
    pacemaker, 66, 81
Activation time, 125
Alternans, 107, 165
Alternating current (AC), 137
Ambulatory (Holter) monitoring,
    147
Amputee, EKG technique, 137
Amyloid, 121
Analogies
    elephant in box, 24
    pathologist / radiologist /
        electrocardiographer, 5
    pennant, 98
    sailboat/vectors, 33
    shadow of scissors, 38
    surgery and EKG, 1
    water skier, 20
Anatomy and physiology, 12
Aneurysm, ventricular, 107, 110
Angina pectoris, 105
Anterior directed forces, 93, 117,
    121
Arrhythmias. See Mechanism,
    disturbances of
Artifacts, 140
    abrupt deflections of baseline, 142
    alternating current, 137, 140
    baseline indistinct, 142
    crossed leads, 143
    damping, 138
    electrode positioning, 143, 147
    loose electrical connection, 156
    muscle tremor, 135, 136, 140
    timing error (50 mm./sec.), 142
    wandering baseline, 136, 140
Artificial pacemaker, 73

Asymmetric hypertrophy, 121
Atria. See also P waves
    anatomy/physiology, 12
    depolarization, 12, 52
    enlargement, 123
    repolarization, 15
Atrial fibrillation, 7, 52
Atrial flutter, 60
Atrial infarct, 122
Atrial tachycardia, 60
Atrioventricular (AV) block. See
    Block, AV
Atrioventricular (AV) node. See
    also Junction, AV, 12
Automaticity, 50
AV diagram, 79
AV junction, 50, 68
AV nodal mechanism. See Junction,
    AV
Axis
    definition, 34, 159
    determination, 34, 159
    deviation, 159, 160

Baseline. See also Artifacts
    definition, 44
Bean, William B., 3
Bidirectional tachycardia, 73
Bigeminy, 74
Bilateral bundle branch block, 95
Biventricular hypertrophy, 133
Blind men and elephant, 22
Block, AV
    definition, 76
    diagram, 79
    first degree, 76
    second degree, 60, 77
        Mobitz, 78

Wenckebach, 78
third degree, 78
Block, bundle branch. See Block, left bundle branch and right bundle branch
Block, entrance, 162
Block, exit, 69
Block, heart. See Block AV
Block, intraventricular. See also Block, left bundle branch and right bundle branch
anterior septal, 93
arborization, 95
bifascicular, 93
combinations, 93, 95
hemiblock (fascicular block)
left anterior, 89
left posterior, 94
miscellaneous forms, 95
parietal, 95
peri-infarction, 95
significance, 97
Block, left bundle branch, 87
and myocardial infarction, 96
and ventricular hypertrophy, 96, 133
subdivisions, 87, 89
Block, right bundle branch, 85
and left anterior hemiblock, 93
and myocardial infarction, 96
and ventricular hypertrophy, 96, 133
incomplete, 87
Block, Sino-atrial (SA), 51, 57
Boundary of potential difference, 15, 108
Bruce test, 151
Bundle branch block. See Block, bundle branch

Calcium, 163, 164
Calibration. See Techniques
Capillary electrometer, 6
Central nervous system, 166
Chamber enlargement. See also specific chamber, 123
Chest lead position, 8, 27
Chloroquine, 163

Combined ventricular hypertrophy, 133
Computer analysis, 10, 157
Concealed conduction, 68
Conduction system, 12
Conduction velocity, 12
Congenital heart disease, 166
Coronary insufficiency, 109
Coronary sinus mechanism. See Junction, mechanism
Coronary sinus node, 13
Crossed leads, 143
Current of injury, 108

Damping, 138
Danger, electrical, 138
Default mechanism, 51
Deflection, definition, 44
Delta wave. See Pre-excitation, ventricular
Description and interpretation of a tracing, 168
Depolarization
anatomy, 12
atrial, 12, 52, 98
boundary of potential difference, 15
compared to condenser, 17
definition, 15, 17
electrical "silence" of inner part of ventricular wall, 110
physiology, 15
Digitalis
acceleration of junction pacemaker, 66
and false positive exercise test, 156
AV block, 163
effect, 161
"PAT with block", 63, 163
toxicity, 163
Diphenylhydantoin, 161
Dissociation
atrial, 58
atrio-ventricular, 55, 81
isorhythmic, 81
longitudinal, in His bundle, 69
Drugs, 161

Dystrophy, muscular, 121

Early repolarization, 110, 128
Echo beats, 69
Ectopic pacemaker. See also
  Mechanism, disturbances of
  definition, 50
Einthoven, Willem
  hypotheses, 7, 26
  triangle, 7, 26
EKG
  definition, 5, 26
  history, 5
  interpretation, 168
  machine, 5, 6, 135
  normal, 44
  perspective, 5
  technique, 135
  vs. ECG, 5
Electrical hazard, 138
Electrocardiographer as consultant,
  5
Electrocardiographic methods, 135
Electrolyte disturbance, 163
Electrometer, capillary, 6
Elephant and blind men, 22
Elephant in a box, 24
Embolism, pulmonary, 164
Emetine, 163
Emphysema, pulmonary, 92, 164
Enlargement. See also
  Hypertrophy, Overload, Strain
  atria, 123
  left ventricle, 124
  right ventricle, 124
Entrance block, 68
Escape beats, 56
Esophageal leads, 148
Exercise test. See also Bruce,
  Master, and graded exercise
  discussion, 149
  false positive/negative, 156
  interpretation, 156
Exit block, 69

F, f waves, 62, 63
Fascicular block. See Block,
  intraventricular

Fetal EKG, 148
Fibrillation
  atrial, 52, 63
  ventricular, 73
First degree AV block, See Block,
  AV
Flutter, atrial, 60
Flutter-fibrillation, 64
Fusion beats, 95

Gain control. See Technique
Galvani, 6
Galvanometer, 6, 26
Goldberger, Emmanuel, 9, 30
Graded exercise tests, 149, 156
Gradient, ventricular. See
  Ventricular gradient
Grant, Robert P., 10
Grounding of EKG machine, See
  Techniques

Harrison, Tinsley, 3
Hazard, electrical, 138
Hemiblock. See Block,
  intraventricular
Herrick, James B., 7
Hexaxial reference system, 31
His, bundle of
  anatomy/physiology, 14
  recording from, 148
History of electrocardiography, 5
Holography, 11
Holter (ambulatory) monitoring,
  148
Horizontal plane reference frame,
  38
Hypercalcemia, 162, 164
Hyperkalemia, 95, 121, 162, 164
Hypertrophy. See also Enlargement
  atrial, see Enlargement
  biventricular, 133
  and bundle branch block, 133
  left ventricular, 126
  right ventricular, 126
  significance, 133
Hypocalcemia, 162, 164
Hypokalemia, 162,164
Hypoxia, 105

Idiopathic cardiac myopathy, 121
Idiopathic hypertrophic subaortic
    stenosis (IHSS), 121
Idioventricular pacemaker, 74
Impulse formation and conduction,
    49, 58
Incomplete right bundle branch
    block, 87
Infarction, myocardial, 113
    accuracy of EKG diagnosis, 119
    anterior, 117
    atrial, 122
    and bundle branch block, 117
    cancellation, 120
    criteria for diagnosis, 113, 115,
        117
    differential diagnosis, 117, 120
    dorsal, 117
    false negative, 122
    false positive, 120
    first description, 7
    inferior, 117
    lateral, 117
    location, 117
    multiple, 122
    old, 119, 120
    PVC, evidence, 119
    recent, 119, 120
    silent, 122
    subendocardial, 117
    technical error, 121
    time for appearance, 122
    transmural, 117
    and WPW syndrome, 82, 121
Injury, myocardial, 107
    current of, 108
    in myocardial infarction, 119
    subendocardial, 108
    subepicardial, 108
    vs. early repolarization, 110
Interference dissociation, 81
Interpretation of electrocardiogram,
    168
Intra-atrial block, 58
Intracardiac recording, 148
Intraventricular block. See Block,
    intraventricular
Intrinsic deflection, 125

Ischemia, myocardial, 105
Isorhythmic dissociation, 66, 81,
    121

J point, 48, 101
Jelly, electrode, 136
Jervell and Lange-Nielsen
    syndrome, 167
Junction, AV
    anatomy/physiology, 12, 68
    mechanisms, 65

Kirchhoff's law, 27

Leads
    atrial, 79
    augmented unipolar, 9, 30
    aVR, aVL, aVF, 30
    bipolar, 8, 26
    chest, positions, 8, 27
    CR, CL, and CF, 8
    definition, 9, 22, 24, 43, 145
    esophageal, 79, 148
    history of, 8
    inspiration, 148
    IV, 8
    IV-F, 8
    orthogonal, 9
    precordial, 8
    standard, 8
    unipolar, 8, 27, 30
    V, 8, 27
    VR, VL, and VF, 29
    why so many, 36
Left anterior hemiblock. See Block,
    intraventricular
Left bundle branch block. See
    Block, left bundle branch
Left posterior hemiblock. See
    Block, intraventricular
Left ventricular hypertrophy. See
    also Enlargement, left ventricular
    discussion, 124
Left ventricular overload, 128
Left ventricular strain, 128
Lewis, Sir Thomas, 7
Lidocaine, 161
Limitations of EKG, 3

Linear conductor, 15
Lown-Ganong-Levine syndrome, 84
Lung disease. See Pulmonary
    disease

Magnesium, 164
Mapping, body surface, 148
Mastectomy, 161
Master test, 150, 154
Mechanism. See also specific names
    analysis, 51
    default, 51, 53, 54
    definition, 47, 49
    disturbances, 56, 57
    escape, 56
    idioventricular, 73
    supraventricular, 50, 68
    usurping, 51, 53
    ventricular, 69
Membrane action potential, 50
Methods, EKG. See also Technique,
    135
Mitral valve prolapse, 107, 121, 156
Mobitz, type II AV block, 78
Monocardiogram, 9
Mononucleosis, 121
Muscle tremor. See Artifacts
Myocardial infarction. See
    Infarction, myocardial

Neurologic disease, 166
Nodal Mechanisms. See Junction,
    AV
Node. See specific node
Non-specific ST-T abnormalities.
    See ST-T complex
Normal EKG, 44
Null plane, 42

Orthogonal reference frame, 31
Osler, Sir William, 4
Overload/strain. See also
    Hypertrophy and Enlargement
    early repolarization, 110
    ventricular, 105, 125, 128

P wave
    definition, 44, 47

genesis, 47, 52
    normal, 47, 52
    "P mitrale", 123
    "P pulmonale", 123
    retrograde, 152
    significance, 98
P, Q, R, S, T, and U. See also under
    individual waves
    definition, 7, 45
    origin of names, 7
PR interval
    definition, 45, 55
    measurement, 55, 172
    normal, 77
    prolonged, 77
P_t wave, 44, 48, 98
Pacemaker, artificial, 74
Pacemaker, wandering atrial. See
    Wandering atrial pacemaker, 53,
    57
Paper speed, 142
Paranodal (or paraspecific) tracts,
    69, 84
Parasystole
    atrial, 60, 75
    ventricular, 75
Parietal block, 95
Paroxysmal atrial tachycardia
    (PAT). See Tachycardia, atrial
"PAT with block", 63
Pectus excavatum, 121
Pericardium
    effusion, 161
    inflammation, 108
Peri-infarction block, 95
Perspective, electrocardiography in,
    5
pH, 164
Pneumothorax, 121
Polarized state, 15
Potassium, 55, 92, 95, 163, 164
Precordial electrode positions, 143
Pre-excitation, ventricular, 82, 121,
    122
Premature atrial contractions
    (PAC), 59
    blocked, 60
Premature ventricular contractions

(PVC), 69
Primary T wave abnormality, 20
Procaine amide, 163
Propranolol, 163
Pulmonary disease, 165
    embolism, 164
    left anterior hemiblock, 165
    P-ST-T pattern, 165
    vs. myocardial infarction, 121,
        165
Purkinje fibers, 14

Q wave
    abnormal, criteria, 115
    abnormal, derivation of, 113
    definition, 45
    normal, 115
Quinidine, 8, 95, 162
QRS complex
    activation time, 125
    amplitude, 47, 126, 160
    analysis, 47
    axis, 34, 159
    contour, 47, 54, 99
    definition, 17, 45
    description, 47, 99
    duration, 47, 54
    frontal projection, 48
    horizontal projection, 48
    measurement, 47
    normal, 47
    orientation, 34, 38, 48
    relation to ST-T, 19
    voltage, 126
QRS-T angle, 101
QS, 45, 115
QT interval
    definition, 48
    long, 162, 164, 167
    short, 162
    syndromes, 167
QX:QT, 151

R wave
    definition, 45
    evidence of infarction, 115
    progression, 115

Rates of various pacemakers, 51, 54
Reciprocal mechanisms, 69
Re-entry, 69
Reference frames
    frontal, 26
    general, 22
    hexaxial, 31
    horizontal, 38
    orthogonal, 9, 31
    three-dimensional concept of
        EKG, 32, 38
    triaxial, 27
Repolarization. See also ST-T
    complex, T wave, P_t, U.
    atrial, 15, 48
    definition, 15, 17
    early, 110
    ventricular, 15, 48, 103
Resistance, skin, 27, 36
Rhythm. See Mechanism
Right bundle branch block. See
    Block, right bundle branch
Right ventricular hypertrophy. See
    Enlargement, right ventricular
Romano-Ward syndrome, 167

S wave, definition, 45
S1, S2, S3, 133
Sarcoid, 121
Secondary T wave abnormality, 20
Sick Sinus Syndrome, 58
Sino-atrial (SA) block. See Block,
    sino-atrial
Sino-ventricular conduction, 51, 58
Sinus
    arrhythmia, 56
    bradycardia, 57
    mechanism, 47, 56
    node, 12
    pause, 56
    tachycardia, 56, 58
Skin resistance. See Resistance, skin
Sodium, 164
Spatial concepts, 38
ST-T complex. See also T wave
    abnormalities, nonspecific, 103
    amplitude, 103, 107

definition, 4, 6, 100
description, 101
discrepancy pattern, 105
dome and dart, 133
early repolarization, 110
high T voltage, 107
instability and clinical
    electrocardiography, 20, 103
low T voltage, 103
nonspecific abnormalities, 103
normal, 48
primary/secondary
    abnormalities, 20, 103
relation to QRS, 19
sensitivity/specificity, 98, 105,
    107
ST segment displacement, 101
ST segment contour, 101
"Standard" leads, 8, 26, 27
Strain, ventricular. See also
    Hypertrophy, Overload, 105, 125,
    128
Stress tests, 149
String galvanometer, 6
Structure and function, 98
Stylus, various types, 142
Subendocardial injury. See Injury,
    Subendocardial
Subepicardial injury. See Injury,
    Subepicardial
Supernormality, 69, 75
Supraventricular mechanism, 50,
    54, 56, 68

T wave. See also ST-T complex
    alternans, 107
    amplitude, 103, 107
    atrial. See P_t wave
    contour, 48
    definition, 17, 46, 100
    description, 100
    high voltage, 107
    low voltage, 103
    nonspecific abnormalities, 103
    normal, 48
    orientation, 34, 48
    primary abnormality, 20, 103

    secondary abnormality, 20, 103
    sensitivity, 20
    tall, 107
T_a wave. See P_t wave
Tachycardia. See also Mechanisms
    and specific tachycardias
    atrial, 60
    atrial with 2° AV block, 60, 63
    bidirectional, 73
    ectopic, 50
    junctional, 65
    "PAT with block", 60, 63
    sinus, 56
    supraventricular, 68
    usurping, 51, 53
    ventricular, 73
Tall T waves, 107
Technique of recording tracings. See
    also Artifacts
    ambulatory (Holter) monitoring,
        147
    amputees, 137
    baseline indistinct, 142
    calibration, 138
    damping, 138
    electrode attachment, 135
    electrode jelly, 136
    electrode positions, 143
    exercise testing, 149
    fetal monitoring, 148
    gain control, 138
    grounding of equipment, 137
    inspiration, deep, lead III, 148
    intracardiac, 148
    labeling the tracing, 140
    mapping, 148
    multichannel recording, 148
    paper speed, 142
    precordial leads, 27, 136, 143
    preparation of patient, 135
    rectilinear conversion, 142
    sensitivity, see Gain control
    stylus adjustment, 142
    tape recording, 147
    telemetry, 10, 147
Telemetry. See Techniques

Tetrahedron, 9
Thioridazine, 161
Third-degree AV block. See Block, AV
Three-dimensional concepts, 38
Timing, errors, 142
Transitional curve, 42
Trauma, 121
Treadmill. See Exercise test
Triangle, Einthoven's, 7
Triaxial reference system, 27

U wave, 21, 46, 101
"Unipolar" leads, 8, 27, 30
Usurping mechanism, 51, 53

V leads, 8, 27
VR, VL, and VF, 29
Vector
    definition, 32
    projection, 32
Vectorcardiogram, 9, 36
Ventricular aberration. See Aberration, ventricular
Ventricular activation time. See Activation time
Ventricular aneurysm. See Aneurysm, ventricular
Ventricular enlargement. See Enlargement, ventricular

Ventricular fibrillation, 73
Ventricular gradient, 19
Ventricular hypertrophy / enlargement / strain / overload, 124, 128
Ventricular mechanisms
    analysis, 53
    escape, 56
    from supraventricular focus, 54
    idioventricular, 54
Ventricular pre-excitation. See Pre-excitation, ventricular
Ventricular strain, 125, 128
Ventricular tachycardia, 73
Voltage
    determinants, 160
    low/high, 161
Volume conductor, 15

Waller, Augustus D., 6
Wandering atrial pacemaker, 53, 57
Waves of the electrocardiogram, 7, 44
Wenckebach, 8, 78
Wilson, Frank N., 2, 8, 27
Wolferth and Wood, 8
Wolff-Parkinson-White syndrome. See also Pre-excitation, 82

X, Y, Z axes, 32